The Respiratory Nursing Handbook

COPD, Asthma, NIV, Bronchiectasis and Breathlessness; A Practical Clinical Guide for Ward, Acute and Community Nurses

Cherry B. Johnston

This book is intended as an educational resource for qualified and student nurses and allied health professionals. It is not a prescribing guide, a diagnostic manual, or a substitute for local clinical policy, formal training, competency assessment, or the judgment of a registered prescriber. Clinical guidance changes. Every guideline position described in this book is named and dated in the text so that the reader can check whether it still stands. Where this book and a current local protocol disagree, the local protocol governs practice. Readers must work within the limits of their own registration, competence, and employer policy at all times.

All case studies in this book are composites. Names are drawn from a fixed roster used across this series and carry no national, ethnic, cultural, or gender significance. Any resemblance to actual patients, clinicians, employers, or institutions is coincidental. Clinical details have been altered so that no individual is identifiable.

The author and publisher make no representations or warranties with respect to the accuracy or completeness of the contents of this work and specifically disclaim all warranties, including without limitation any implied warranties of fitness for a particular purpose. Neither the author nor the publisher shall be liable for any loss of profit or any other commercial damages, nor for any injury, loss, or damage alleged to arise directly or indirectly from the use or application of any content in this book. The reader assumes full responsibility for clinical decisions taken in practice.

First edition, 2026.

ISBN; 979-8-90599-853-9

Staten House

Table of Contents

Preface

This book began with a question that has an uncomfortable answer.

Ask a group of respiratory nurses how confident they feel teaching a patient to use an inhaler. Most will say confident. Then ask them to demonstrate the eight devices their unit actually stocks. In one specialised respiratory inpatient unit, researchers did exactly that. Eighty four percent of the nurses described themselves as moderately or extremely confident about delivering inhaler education. Their mean score for correct steps across the devices was 47 percent, and confidence showed no relationship at all to competence (Swami et al., 2021).

That finding is not an indictment of nurses. It is an indictment of how respiratory care gets taught. The knowledge exists. It sits in guidelines that run to ninety pages, in confidential enquiry reports written for service directors, in journal supplements that nobody reads at three in the morning. What is missing is the layer in between: the working translation that tells a nurse standing at the end of a bed what to do next, and why, and when to stop and call someone.

Consider the pattern across three separate national investigations. The 2014 National Review of Asthma Deaths found potentially preventable factors in two thirds of the records it scrutinised, and judged overall asthma management to be good in fewer than one fifth of the people who died (Royal College of Physicians, 2014). The 2017 confidential enquiry into acute noninvasive ventilation concluded that care had been suboptimal in more than 80 percent of the cases reviewed (National Confidential Enquiry into Patient Outcome and Death, 2017). British Thoracic Society oxygen audits have repeatedly found that a large minority of patients receiving oxygen have no prescription for it, and that a large minority of those who do have one have no target saturation range specified (O'Driscoll et al., 2017).

Three investigations. Three different conditions. The same finding underneath all of them, which is that the failure is rarely a failure of knowledge at the level of the specialist. It is a failure of translation at the level of the ward.

This handbook is organised around that gap. It is not arranged by disease, which is how reference books are arranged, and which works beautifully for the reader who already knows what she is looking for. It is arranged by clinical moment. The first ten minutes. The first hour. The decision to escalate. The conversation nobody trained you for. A nurse who does not yet know what she is looking at cannot use an index, because an index requires her to already have the answer she is trying to find.

Six chapters cover the conditions that fill respiratory and acute medical beds. Three consecutive chapters cover noninvasive ventilation, because setting it up, rescuing it, and recognising when it has become a form of prolonged dying are three different problems that a single chapter cannot hold. Two chapters cover breathlessness, because it is the symptom where nursing outperforms medicine and the one for which nurses receive the least preparation. The remaining chapters cover oxygen, blood gases, procedures, and the discharge that determines whether the patient comes back in eleven days.

A word about currency. Respiratory guidance moved substantially between 2023 and 2025. The Global Initiative for Chronic Obstructive Lung Disease replaced its four group assessment tool with a three group version built around exacerbation history. The British Thoracic Society, the National Institute for Health and Care Excellence, and the Scottish Intercollegiate Guidelines Network published a joint asthma guideline that withdrew the recommendation for short acting reliever therapy used alone. Anyone trained before those changes is now working from a map that no longer matches the ground. Where this book states a guideline position, it names the body and the year, so that the reader can check what has happened since.

Every chapter ends with something to do rather than something to think about. Some of those actions will be uncomfortable. The inhaler chapter asks you to score your own technique before you read the teaching section, and most readers will not enjoy the result. That discomfort is the point. Confidence that has never been tested is not confidence. It is a habit.

One final note on scope. This book supports practice. It does not authorise it. Ventilator settings, drug doses, and escalation thresholds are described here at the level of published national guidance so that a nurse understands what is happening and why, not so that she can act outside her competence or her local protocol. The difference between understanding a decision and being the person who makes it matters, and it matters most in exactly the situations this book describes.

Cherry Johnston is a registered nurse currently working in respiratory care.

PART I: THE FOUNDATIONS OF RESPIRATORY ASSESSMENT

Chapter 1: Reading the Breathless Patient

Chapter Complexity Level: Foundational

Prerequisites: None. This chapter assumes no prior respiratory experience.

Time Investment: Forty five minutes to read. Three shifts to embed.

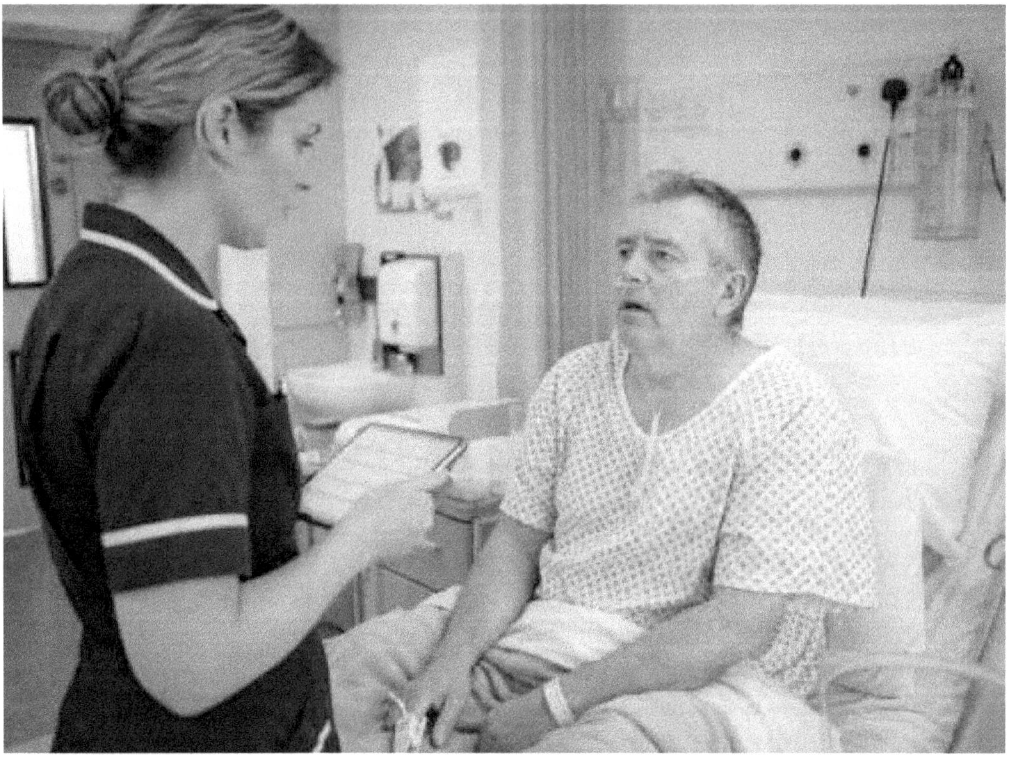

Every nurse on every ward records a respiratory rate. It takes fifteen seconds, it goes in the same box on the same chart it has occupied for a decade, and it is the observation on that chart most likely to be wrong. Not wrong by a little. Wrong by a pattern, recorded as 18 or 20 or 16 because those are the numbers that appear when nobody actually counted. The respiratory rate is also the earliest and most sensitive marker of physiological deterioration available at the bedside. Both statements have been true for years, and they sit side by side on millions of observation charts. This chapter is about the gap between them.

1.1 What Assessment Actually Means

Respiratory assessment is not a set of observations. It is a judgment about trajectory, and the observations are the raw material.

The distinction matters because a nurse who is collecting numbers will record a saturation of 89 percent and move on to the next bay. A nurse who is judging trajectory will record the same number and immediately ask three further questions. What was it yesterday. What is the patient doing to achieve it. What happens if I do nothing for an hour.

Respiratory assessment, defined usefully rather than formally, is the process of establishing how hard a patient is working to maintain gas exchange, and whether that effort is sustainable. Gas exchange is the outcome. Work is the cost. Most bedside errors in respiratory nursing come from measuring the outcome and ignoring the cost.

A patient with saturations of 94 percent who is using accessory muscles, speaking in short phrases, and sitting bolt upright is in more danger than a patient with saturations of 89 percent who is chatting comfortably at their usual baseline. The oximeter cannot tell you which is which. It reports a number that has already been paid for, without telling you the price.

1.2 The Number Everyone Records

Respiratory rate earned its place in early warning scores for a straightforward physiological reason. Ventilation is the body's fastest available compensation. When metabolic demand rises, when acid accumulates, when cardiac output falls, breathing changes before blood pressure does and long before consciousness does.

That sensitivity is precisely why the measurement is fragile. A rate counted for 15 seconds and multiplied by four carries a margin of error of plus or minus four breaths, which is the difference between a score of zero and a score of two on most track and trigger systems. A rate estimated by glancing at a chest for a moment carries a margin of error nobody has measured, because nobody can.

Count for a full 60 seconds while appearing to do something else. Take the radial pulse and keep your fingers there after you have finished counting it. Patients who know their breathing is being watched change their breathing. This is not deception, and it is not a trick. It is the same reason blood pressure gets measured after the patient has been seated quietly.

> **Teaching Point:** *A respiratory rate of 20 recorded four times in a row is not stability. It is very often a nurse who did not count. Look for identical repeated values across a chart as a marker of measurement failure, not of a settled patient.*

1.3 A Sequence That Holds

Under pressure, people revert to whatever sequence they have practised. If no sequence has been practised, they revert to whatever they saw last. The following order takes about ten minutes and works because it moves from what you can see across the room to what requires equipment.

Begin from the doorway, before touching anything. Position tells you most of it. A patient sitting forward with hands braced on their thighs or on a table has adopted the tripod position, which increases the mechanical advantage of the accessory muscles. Nobody adopts it for comfort. A patient lying flat and breathing quietly is rarely in acute respiratory difficulty, though they may still be profoundly unwell for other reasons.

Then listen to speech. Speech is a free lung function test and it costs nothing. Full sentences, short sentences, phrases, single words, no words. That scale takes two seconds to apply and it correlates with severity across every condition in this book.

Then look at the work. Accessory muscle use at the neck and shoulders. Intercostal or subcostal recession. Nasal flaring. Pursed lip breathing, which is a learned compensation in chronic obstructive disease and tells you something about how long this patient has been managing. Note whether expiration is prolonged, which points toward airflow obstruction, or whether breathing is rapid and shallow, which points more toward restrictive disease or pain.

Then colour and consciousness. Central cyanosis, assessed at the lips and tongue rather than the fingers, is a late sign and an unreliable one, particularly in anaemia and in patients with darker skin tones. Drowsiness in a breathless patient is the observation that should stop you where you stand. In a patient with obstructive disease it may indicate carbon dioxide retention rather than fatigue, and it is discussed in detail in section 3.4.

Only then reach for equipment. By this point you already know most of what the equipment is going to tell you, and you know something it cannot tell you at all. Saturations, and crucially the oxygen the patient is receiving to achieve them, because a saturation without a corresponding inspired oxygen concentration is meaningless. Respiratory rate, counted properly. Then auscultation, if you have it.

For the nurse who is not a specialist, four findings on auscultation are worth distinguishing reliably, and the rest can wait. Wheeze, which is expiratory and musical and indicates narrowed airways. Coarse crackles, which shift or clear with coughing and suggest secretions. Fine crackles, which do not clear and appear at the lung bases in fibrosis and pulmonary oedema. And the absence of breath sounds over a region, which in a distressed patient is the most urgent finding on this list.

1.4 What Gets Misread

Three assessment errors recur often enough to be worth naming.

The first is treating the oximeter as the assessment rather than as one input to it. Pulse oximetry is degraded by poor peripheral perfusion, movement, nail varnish, and cold hands, and it says nothing whatsoever about carbon dioxide. A patient can have a saturation of 96 percent and a dangerously high carbon dioxide level at the same moment. In fact, if that saturation was achieved with generous supplemental oxygen in a patient prone to hypercapnia, the two findings are related.

The second is the use of the wrong early warning scale. Most track and trigger systems in the United Kingdom contain a second oxygen saturation scale intended for patients with a documented risk of hypercapnic respiratory failure and a target range of 88 to 92 percent. It has to be prescribed by a doctor to be used. Applying the standard scale to such a patient generates false alarm at their normal state. Applying the alternative scale to a patient who does not qualify generates false reassurance while they deteriorate, which is the more dangerous error of the two.

The third is mistaking a settled appearance for a settled patient. Exhaustion looks calm. A respiratory rate that falls from 34 to 22 in a patient who is becoming drowsy is not improvement, and the chart will not tell you which of those two things has happened. Only the sequence in section 1.3 will.

1.5 Assessment Under Pressure

The following account is a composite, with details changed for anonymity.

Wren had been qualified for seven months when she took the handover for bay three. The patient in bed 11 was described as stable, admitted two days earlier with an infective exacerbation of chronic obstructive pulmonary disease, saturations 90 to 92 percent, for discharge planning in the morning.

At the 2 a.m. observation round she recorded saturations of 91 percent and a respiratory rate of 20. Both were within range. Both matched the previous three sets exactly. She almost moved on.

What stopped her was not a number. It was that the patient had stopped talking. On the previous round he had complained about the tea. Now he answered in single words and did not open his eyes fully between them. His saturations were unchanged because he was on 4 litres via nasal cannulae and had been all night.

She escalated, and the initial response was reasonable and wrong. The registrar reviewed the chart remotely, saw four sets of observations with no change, and asked her to repeat them in an hour. Wren said something that she later described as the most useful sentence she had learned in seven months, which was that the numbers had not changed but the patient had, and that she thought he was retaining carbon dioxide. A blood gas taken 20 minutes later showed a pH of 7.26 and a markedly raised carbon dioxide level.

What made the difference was not knowledge she did not have. It was that she had a sequence, and the sequence contained an item that the observation chart does not: speech. The chart had no box for the fact that a man who had been complaining about the tea had stopped forming sentences.

The complication worth noting is that the previous three sets of observations had almost certainly been inaccurate. A respiratory rate of 20 recorded identically three times across a night is the signature described in section 1.2. Had those rates been counted properly, the trajectory would have been visible several hours earlier, and the conversation with the registrar would not have needed to be won.

Teaching points:

Escalation succeeds when it reports a change rather than a value. A number within range is not an argument, but a described difference between two points in time is.

Any observation set that exactly repeats the previous one deserves suspicion before it deserves reassurance.

1.6 The Same Numbers Twice

The following are composite cases.

Case A

Tatum, aged 71, arrived on the acute medical unit with saturations of 88 percent on air and a respiratory rate of 26. She was assessed from the doorway by a nurse who noted that she was sitting forward, speaking in short phrases, and using neck muscles. Oxygen was started at a target range of 88 to 92 percent, an arterial blood gas was requested within 15 minutes, and the medical team was told that this was a patient who looked like she was working hard. She was reviewed within the half hour.

Case B

Hollis, aged 68, arrived the same evening with saturations of 88 percent on air and a respiratory rate of 26. He was recorded, scored, and placed in the queue for medical review. He was comfortable, lying back, and answering in full sentences. He was seen two hours later. Nothing was missed, because there was nothing to miss.

The two patients produced identical numbers. What separated them was work of breathing, which no observation chart captures and which the sequence in section 1.3 captures in the first ten seconds. Tatum was paying a high metabolic price for 88 percent. Hollis was not, because 88 percent was close to his usual baseline and he was making no unusual effort to hold it. Prioritisation between two apparently identical patients rests almost entirely on evidence gathered before the equipment comes out.

The Working Knowledge

Start here. Respiratory assessment measures effort, not just result, and the observation chart records result almost exclusively. That single asymmetry accounts for a large share of missed deterioration on general wards.

Build on it. Effort is visible from the doorway, in position, speech, and accessory muscle use, which means the most informative part of a respiratory assessment happens before any equipment is touched and costs nothing but attention.

Then add this. Because effort is where the information is, the numbers on the chart are only interpretable against a trajectory. A saturation of 91 percent means one thing in a patient who has always run at 91, and something entirely different in a patient who was 96 percent yesterday and is now working to hold 91. The same logic applies to a falling respiratory rate, which is improvement in a patient who is brightening and a terminal sign in a patient who is tiring.

That sequence changes what escalation sounds like. A nurse who reports a value invites the response that the value is acceptable. A nurse who reports a change, anchored in something specific that was true earlier and is not true now, is describing a trajectory, and trajectories are what clinicians act on. Wren's registrar did not respond to a saturation of 91 percent. He responded to a man who had stopped forming sentences.

Chapter 1 Review Questions

1. **A patient with known COPD has saturations of 90 percent, a respiratory rate of 22, is sitting forward with hands braced on a table, and answers in three word phrases. The previous set of observations two hours ago recorded saturations of 91 percent and a respiratory rate of 20. What is the most appropriate interpretation?**

A) The patient is stable because the saturations have changed by only one percentage point

B) The patient is compensating at a high metabolic cost and needs prompt review

C) The patient requires an immediate increase in oxygen flow rate

D) The observations should be repeated in a further two hours

Answer: B. The saturation change is trivial and the work of breathing is not. Tripod positioning and three word phrases both indicate substantial respiratory effort. Option C is unsafe because increasing oxygen without a target range and a blood gas risks worsening hypercapnia in a patient with COPD, as discussed in Chapter 2.

2. **Which of the following most reliably indicates that a recorded respiratory rate may be inaccurate?**

A) A rate above 30 in a patient who appears comfortable

B) A rate of 20 recorded identically across three consecutive observation sets

C) A rate that differs from the rate recorded by the previous shift

D) A rate recorded at the same time as the blood pressure

Answer: B. Identical repeated values are a recognised signature of estimation rather than measurement. A rate that changes between shifts is expected and is not in itself suspicious.

3. **A breathless patient with COPD becomes drowsy while saturations remain at 92 percent on 4 litres via nasal cannulae. What does this most likely indicate?**

A) The patient is settling and should be allowed to rest

B) The oxygen concentration is inadequate and should be increased

C) Possible carbon dioxide retention requiring urgent blood gas analysis

D) Normal overnight variation in conscious level

Answer: C. Saturations report oxygenation only and are silent on carbon dioxide. Drowsiness in a breathless patient with obstructive disease should be treated as possible hypercapnia until a blood gas excludes it. Option B would worsen the situation.

Chapter 2: Oxygen as a Drug

Chapter Complexity Level: Foundational

Prerequisites: Chapter 1. Familiarity with your local oxygen prescription chart.

Time Investment: Fifty minutes to read. One shift to audit.

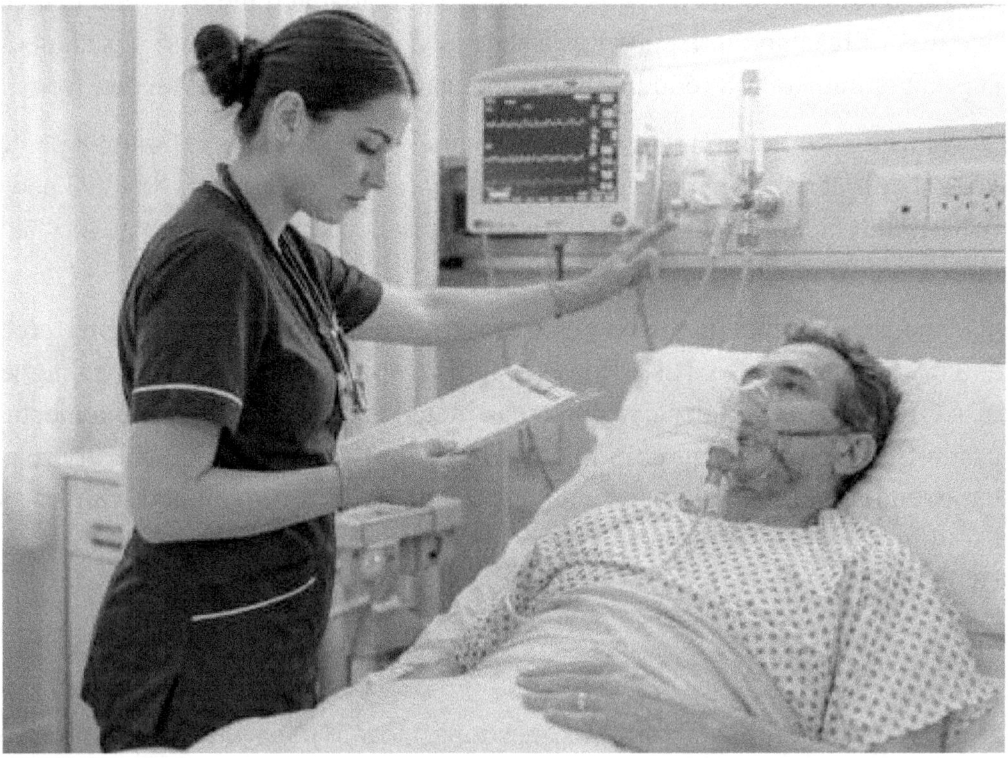

In the 2015 British Thoracic Society national oxygen audit, 42 percent of patients receiving oxygen in United Kingdom hospitals had no oxygen prescription at all, and among those who did, a target saturation range was frequently absent. A third of patients were outside their intended saturation range, with roughly twice as many above it as below it (O'Driscoll et al., 2017). The figure that should unsettle a respiratory nurse is not the missing prescriptions. It is the direction of the error. More patients were receiving too much oxygen than too little, in a country that has been auditing this since 2008.

2.1 What a Prescription Requires

Oxygen is a drug. It is stocked, it is administered, it is titrated, and it causes harm at the wrong dose. It is also the only drug on most wards that any member of staff can turn up without recording anything.

A valid oxygen prescription has three components, and a prescription missing any of them is not a prescription. It specifies a target saturation range rather than a flow rate, because the range is the therapeutic goal and the flow rate is merely one way of reaching it. It specifies a starting delivery device. And it is signed for at each administration round, in the same way any other drug is signed for.

The target saturation range for most acutely unwell adults is 94 to 98 percent. For patients at risk of hypercapnic respiratory failure, the range is 88 to 92 percent (O'Driscoll et al., 2017). Those two ranges account for nearly every adult inpatient a ward nurse will meet.

The second range is the one that causes anxiety, so it is worth being precise about who it applies to. Risk of hypercapnic respiratory failure is not a diagnosis of COPD. It is a broader category that includes severe COPD, bronchiectasis, cystic fibrosis, chest wall deformity, neuromuscular disease, and obesity related hypoventilation. A patient over 50 who is a long term smoker with chronic breathlessness and no confirmed diagnosis should be managed as presumed COPD until proven otherwise.

2.2 Choosing the Device

Device selection follows from two questions. How hypoxaemic is the patient, and does the delivered concentration need to be predictable.

Variable performance devices, which include nasal cannulae and simple face masks, deliver a concentration that changes with the patient's own inspiratory flow. A breathless patient with a high peak inspiratory flow entrains more room air and receives a lower effective concentration than the same device would deliver to a settled patient. That variability is acceptable in a patient whose target range is 94 to 98 percent. It is a problem in a patient whose safe window is four percentage points wide.

Fixed performance devices, principally Venturi masks, deliver a set concentration regardless of inspiratory effort, provided the flow rate marked on the valve is used. That predictability is the entire reason they exist and the reason they belong on patients at risk of hypercapnia.

Device	Typical flow	Approximate delivered oxygen	Best suited to
Nasal cannulae	1 to 6 L per minute	24 to 40 percent, variable	Mild hypoxaemia, patients who need to eat and talk
Simple face mask	5 to 10 L per minute	40 to 60 percent, variable	Moderate hypoxaemia, no hypercapnia risk
Venturi mask	Flow marked on each valve	24, 28, 31, 35, 40 or 60 percent, fixed	Any patient at risk of hypercapnic respiratory failure
Reservoir mask	15 L per minute	60 to 80 percent or higher	Critical illness, saturations below 85 percent, peri arrest

Two practical points defeat this table more often than any theoretical objection. A simple face mask run below 5 litres per minute allows exhaled carbon dioxide to accumulate inside the mask and be rebreathed, so it must never be used at low flow. And a Venturi valve set to the wrong flow rate stops being a fixed performance device altogether, which makes the number printed on the valve one of the most important numbers on the bed space.

> **Teaching Point:** *The commonest oxygen error on a general ward is not the flow rate. It is the absence of a documented target range, which leaves every subsequent decision, including yours, without a reference point.*

2.3 Titration in Practice

The following worked example uses a composite case.

Garnet, aged 74, is admitted overnight with breathlessness and a productive cough. He has a 40 pack year smoking history and no formal COPD diagnosis. He arrives from the emergency department on a reservoir mask at 15 litres per minute with saturations of 99 percent. There is no oxygen prescription on the chart.

Step one, what the situation actually is. A saturation of 99 percent is not a reassuring number. In a patient of this age and smoking history it is a warning, because it indicates that oxygen is being delivered far in excess of any plausible therapeutic target and that the risk of hypercapnia has not been considered.

Step two, what to do before anything else. The instinct is to reduce the oxygen immediately. The better first action is to obtain a blood gas and a prescription, because the safe target range depends on the carbon dioxide level and on whether this patient has previously required ventilatory support. Reducing oxygen abruptly in a patient whose true oxygenation is unknown risks a rapid fall in saturation.

Step three, the interim position. Pending gases, guidance supports aiming for 88 to 92 percent in patients with risk factors for hypercapnia but no history of respiratory acidosis, using a 24 percent Venturi mask at 2 to 3 litres per minute, a 28 percent mask at 4 litres, or nasal cannulae at 1 to 2 litres (O'Driscoll et al., 2017). The nurse's role here is to move the patient from an unpredictable high concentration onto a predictable low one and to monitor closely while doing it.

The complicating moment. The night registrar declines to prescribe a target range on the grounds that Garnet has no confirmed COPD diagnosis and should be treated as a standard patient at 94 to 98 percent. This is a defensible clinical position and it is also the exact scenario the guidance anticipates. The resolution is not to argue about the diagnosis. It is to ask for the blood gas, which converts an argument about labels into a decision about numbers. Garnet's gas returns with a carbon dioxide level in the normal range, and the target is set at 94 to 98 percent with a documented note to review if his carbon dioxide rises.

What this example shows. The nurse changed the outcome twice. She converted an unprescribed situation into a prescribed one, and she converted a disagreement about a diagnosis into a request for data. Neither action required her to override a prescriber, and neither required specialist knowledge.

2.4 When Oxygen Causes Harm

Excess oxygen harms patients through two distinct mechanisms, and conflating them causes confusion.

The first mechanism is hypercapnia in susceptible patients. High concentrations of oxygen worsen carbon dioxide retention through several routes, the most significant of which is increased dead space ventilation as hypoxic pulmonary vasoconstriction is released and blood is redirected to poorly ventilated lung units. The result is a rising carbon dioxide level, a falling pH, and eventually a reduction in conscious level. This is a real and rapid danger and it is the reason the 88 to 92 percent range exists.

The second mechanism applies to everybody. Liberal oxygen in acutely unwell patients who are not hypoxaemic is associated with increased mortality across a range of conditions (Chu et al., 2018). This finding surprised the field when it was published and it has changed practice in stroke and myocardial infarction in particular, where routine oxygen for non hypoxaemic patients is no longer recommended.

The practical consequence is a single rule that covers both mechanisms. Oxygen treats hypoxaemia. It does not treat breathlessness, anxiety, or a low reading on a poorly attached probe, and giving it for those reasons is not neutral.

2.5 How Often to Look

Titration is worthless without a monitoring interval attached to it, and monitoring intervals are the part of oxygen therapy most often left to habit.

Any change in oxygen concentration invalidates the previous set of observations. After an increase or a decrease, saturations need rechecking within five minutes to confirm the direction of travel, and a patient at risk of hypercapnia needs a blood gas within 30 to 60 minutes of any significant increase in delivered oxygen (O'Driscoll et al., 2017). A saturation checked immediately after a change tells you about the probe. A saturation checked at five minutes tells you about the patient.

Frequency between changes should follow the patient's early warning score rather than the ward's routine. A patient scoring highly on a track and trigger system who is checked four hourly because that is the ward's default has been assigned a monitoring interval by the drug round, not by their physiology.

Two further habits are worth building. Never remove oxygen to obtain a room air saturation in a patient who clearly requires it, a practice that persists in some units and serves no purpose that a documented inspired concentration does not serve better. And record the delivery device alongside the saturation every time. A saturation of 92 percent on 24 percent Venturi and a saturation of 92 percent on 15 litres via reservoir mask describe two entirely different patients, and a chart that does not distinguish them is not a record.

Humidification deserves a brief mention because it is frequently requested and rarely necessary at low flows. Nasal cannulae at up to 4 litres per minute do not routinely require humidification. Higher flows, long term use, and patients with tenacious secretions or an artificial airway are a different matter, and the bronchiectasis considerations in Chapter 11 apply.

2.6 The Conversation About an Unprescribed Prescription

The following account is a composite, with details changed for anonymity.

Indigo had been a Band 5 on a respiratory ward for 14 months when she found a post operative patient on nasal cannulae at 3 litres per minute with no prescription, no documented indication, and saturations of 97 percent. The oxygen had been running for six days. Nobody could say who had started it.

Her first approach failed. She raised it on the ward round as a documentation issue, and it was received as one. The consultant agreed it should be written up, the team moved on, and nothing changed for a further two days.

Her second approach worked, and the difference was framing. She asked the same consultant whether the patient still needed oxygen at all, and pointed out that his saturations had been 96 to 98 percent for four days and that nobody had trialled him without it. That reframing converted a paperwork problem into a clinical question, and clinical questions get answered on ward rounds. The oxygen was stopped that morning. The patient maintained 96 percent on air.

What is worth extracting from this is not that Indigo was persistent. It is that a request to complete a chart and a request to review a treatment are heard completely differently, even when they concern exactly the same patient. Section 2.1 described the components of a valid prescription. The reason those components matter clinically, rather than administratively, is that they force somebody to decide what the oxygen is for.

Teaching points:

Framing an oxygen issue as a documentation gap invites a documentation response, which does not change what the patient receives.

Oxygen that nobody started and nobody stopped is common in surgical and older adult wards, and a saturation comfortably above target is the signal to look for it.

The Practitioner's Bottom Line

The practical position is narrower than the guideline that supports it. Find the target range before you touch the flow meter, and if there is no range documented, that absence is the clinical problem you have just discovered, not an obstacle to the one you were looking for.

For patients at risk of hypercapnic respiratory failure, move to a fixed performance device early and check that the flow rate matches the number on the valve. That single habit prevents more harm than any amount of theoretical understanding of hypoxic drive, a concept that is more often invoked than correctly applied and that explains less of the physiology than the dead space mechanism described in section 2.4.

Treat a saturation that sits comfortably above the target range as an abnormal result. It is the finding most likely to be ignored on a ward round and the one most likely to indicate that nobody has thought about this patient's oxygen since admission.

And when you escalate, ask what the oxygen is for. Not whether it has been written up. The audit evidence has been consistent for well over a decade, which suggests the problem is not that clinicians do not know the guidance. It is that unprescribed oxygen rarely presents itself as a clinical question, and it takes a nurse at the bedside to convert it into one.

Chapter 2 Review Questions

1. **A patient with severe COPD and a documented target range of 88 to 92 percent has saturations of 97 percent on a 28 percent Venturi mask. What is the most appropriate immediate action?**

A) Continue, because saturations above target are not harmful

B) Change to nasal cannulae at the same flow rate

C) Reduce the delivered oxygen concentration and recheck saturations, escalating for review of the prescription

D) Stop oxygen entirely and reassess in one hour

Answer: C. Saturations above target in a patient at risk of hypercapnia require the concentration to be stepped down toward the intended range, with monitoring. Option D risks an abrupt fall in oxygenation. Option B replaces a fixed performance device with a variable one, which is the wrong direction for this patient.

2. **Why must a simple face mask never be run below 5 litres per minute?**

A) The mask will not seal adequately at lower flows

B) Exhaled carbon dioxide accumulates within the mask and is rebreathed

C) The delivered oxygen concentration becomes fixed rather than variable

D) The humidification system fails below this threshold

Answer: B. Flow must be sufficient to flush expired gas from the mask. This is a design characteristic of the device rather than a comfort issue.

3. **Which statement best describes the relationship between oxygen and breathlessness?**

A) Oxygen relieves breathlessness in most patients regardless of saturation

B) Oxygen treats hypoxaemia and does not reliably relieve breathlessness in patients who are not hypoxaemic

C) Oxygen should be given to any patient reporting breathlessness pending assessment

D) Breathlessness is a more reliable indicator of hypoxaemia than pulse oximetry

Answer: B. Breathlessness and hypoxaemia are distinct. Non pharmacological approaches to breathlessness in non hypoxaemic patients are covered in Chapter 13.

Chapter 3: Blood Gases Without Panic

Chapter Complexity Level: Foundational

Prerequisites: Chapters 1 and 2.

Time Investment: One hour to read. Twelve worked gases to practise.

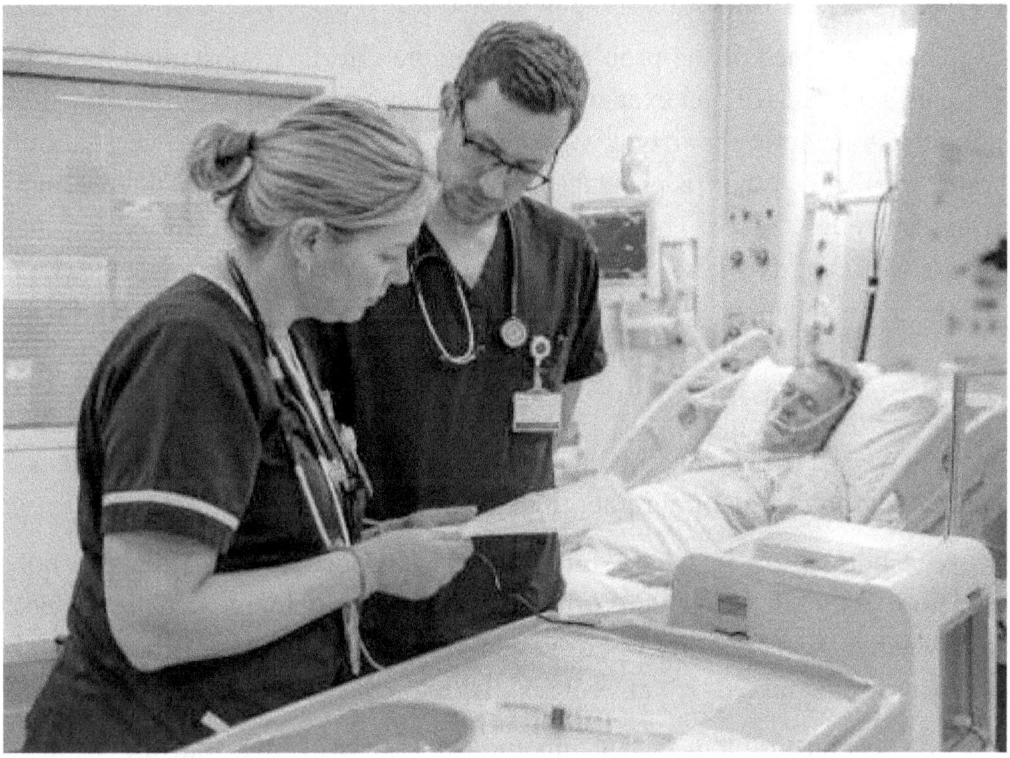

The printout is about the size of a supermarket receipt. It comes out of the analyser warm, curls slightly at the edges, and contains roughly 20 values of which four matter for the decision in front of you. Most nurses receive it, glance at it, and hand it to a doctor. That handover takes four seconds and it is where a great deal of respiratory nursing quietly stops. The reason is not that blood gas interpretation is difficult. It is that almost nobody is taught it as a sequence, and a value without a sequence is just a number on a warm piece of paper.

3.1 The Problem With Gases

Arterial blood gas interpretation has a peculiar status in nursing education. It appears in every respiratory course. It is examined, revised, and forgotten within weeks, and the reason it is forgotten is that it is usually taught as a classification exercise rather than as a clinical decision.

A nurse who can correctly label a gas as compensated respiratory acidosis has achieved something, but not the thing that matters at two in the morning. The clinically useful question is narrower. Does this patient need ventilatory support, do they need it now, and what is the trend.

The prevalence of the problem justifies the effort. A substantial minority of patients admitted with an exacerbation of chronic obstructive pulmonary disease are already acidotic on arrival, which is why acute noninvasive ventilation is a ward level rather than a critical care level treatment in the United Kingdom (Davidson et al., 2016). Those patients arrive already in the territory this chapter covers, onto wards where the nurse is the person who will be present when the second gas is taken.

3.2 Why Mnemonics Fail

Most nurses have been taught a mnemonic. Most cannot apply it under pressure, and the reason is structural rather than personal.

Mnemonics for acid base interpretation encode the classification, not the decision. They tell you which of four boxes a result belongs in. They do not tell you whether the patient in front of you is deteriorating, and they collapse entirely when a result is mixed, which real results frequently are.

The second problem is that mnemonics start with pH. Starting with pH is defensible in a physiology examination and unhelpful at the bedside, because it front loads the abstract quantity and postpones the one that determines your immediate action, which is oxygenation.

The approach in section 3.3 reverses that order deliberately. It asks the questions in the order in which the answers change what you do.

3.3 A Sequence of Four Questions

Ask these four questions in this order, every time, on every gas, including the ones that look normal.

First, is the patient oxygenated? Look at the oxygen level and, critically, at the inspired oxygen concentration it was achieved on. A normal oxygen level on 60 percent oxygen is not a normal result. It is a compensated one, and it tells you how much support is being spent to hold the number where it is. This is the same asymmetry between result and effort described in section 1.1, expressed in different units.

Second, what is the pH? Below 7.35 is acidosis. Above 7.45 is alkalosis. The degree matters more than the label. A pH of 7.34 and a pH of 7.21 are both acidosis and they belong to different clinical urgencies entirely.

Third, is the carbon dioxide explaining the pH? If the pH is low and the carbon dioxide is high, the problem is ventilation. The patient is not clearing carbon dioxide adequately, and the treatment for that is ventilatory support rather than oxygen. If the pH is low and the carbon dioxide is low or normal, the acidosis has a metabolic cause and the raised respiratory rate is compensation rather than pathology.

Fourth, how long has this been going on? The bicarbonate answers this, and it is the value nurses most often skip. Bicarbonate rises slowly, over days, as the kidneys retain base to buffer a chronically raised carbon dioxide. A high carbon dioxide with a high bicarbonate and a near normal pH describes a patient who has been living in this state for some time. A high carbon dioxide with a normal bicarbonate and a low pH describes something that has happened recently, and recent is the word that changes the urgency.

> **Teaching Point:** *The bicarbonate is the clock. Carbon dioxide tells you the current problem, and bicarbonate tells you roughly how long the body has had to prepare for it.*

3.4 Acute and Chronic Retention

The distinction between acute and chronic hypercapnia is the single most useful thing in this chapter, and it is the distinction most often lost in a handover.

A patient with long standing severe COPD may live with a carbon dioxide level well above the normal range and a pH within normal limits, sustained by a raised bicarbonate. That patient is not in respiratory failure at that moment. Their gas looks alarming and their clinical state is stable, and treating the number rather than the patient leads to unnecessary intervention.

The same patient during an exacerbation develops a further rise in carbon dioxide on top of the chronic elevation. The kidneys cannot compensate at that speed, so the pH falls. It is the falling pH, not the absolute carbon dioxide level, that identifies acute deterioration and that determines whether noninvasive ventilation is indicated (Davidson et al., 2016).

This has a direct nursing consequence. A carbon dioxide value reported in isolation at handover is close to useless. A carbon dioxide value reported alongside the pH and the bicarbonate describes a trajectory. Chapter 8 returns to the specific thresholds that trigger ventilatory support, but the underlying logic is established here.

There is also a common trap in the other direction. A patient with chronic retention who receives generous supplemental oxygen may develop a rising carbon dioxide with a falling pH over a period of hours, having arrived comfortable. The gas taken on admission was reassuring. The gas taken at 4 a.m. is not, and the intervening variable was the oxygen described in Chapter 2.

3.5 Working Through a Gas

The following worked example uses a composite case.

Calloway, aged 66, has COPD and is admitted with three days of increasing breathlessness and green sputum. She is on a 28 percent Venturi mask. The gas shows a pH of 7.29, a carbon dioxide of 8.4 kilopascals, an oxygen level of 7.1 kilopascals, and a bicarbonate of 31 millimoles per litre.

Step one, oxygenation. The oxygen level is low for a patient receiving 28 percent oxygen. She is hypoxaemic despite supplementation, though her saturations are within the 88 to 92 percent target. Both facts can be true, and the saturation alone would not have revealed the first.

Step two, pH. At 7.29 she is acidotic, and meaningfully so rather than marginally.

Step three, carbon dioxide. At 8.4 it is clearly raised, and it explains the acidosis. This is a ventilatory problem.

Step four, bicarbonate. At 31 it is raised, which indicates renal compensation established over days or longer. She has chronic retention.

Putting it together. Calloway has acute on chronic hypercapnic respiratory failure. The raised bicarbonate shows she has been retaining carbon dioxide for some time. The low pH shows that something has changed recently and that compensation is now inadequate. This combination is the classic indication for noninvasive ventilation.

The complicating moment. The obvious action is to request noninvasive ventilation immediately. That is not quite the correct next step. Guidance is explicit that standard medical therapy comes first, including controlled oxygen, bronchodilators, steroids and antibiotics, because a proportion of patients presenting with acidosis correct within the first hour on these measures alone. The correct action is to ensure optimal medical therapy is delivered, alert the team that this patient meets the criteria if she does not improve, and repeat the gas within an hour. The nurse who insists on immediate ventilation and the nurse who waits four hours for the next routine gas have both made an error, and the second error is more common.

What this shows. The four questions produced the diagnosis in under a minute. What they did not produce, and could not, was the timing decision. That came from knowing what happens in the first hour, which is the subject of Chapter 8.

3.6 A Gas That Misleads

The following is a composite case; identifying details have been changed.

Background

Merritt, aged 58, was admitted through the emergency department with breathlessness and chest tightness. She had a history of anxiety and no diagnosed respiratory disease. She had attended twice in the preceding year with similar symptoms and had been discharged both times.

Presentation

She was distressed, tachypnoeic at 32 breaths per minute, speaking in short sentences, with saturations of 96 percent on air. She described tingling in her hands. The initial impression recorded in the notes was hyperventilation secondary to anxiety.

Analysis

The blood gas showed a pH of 7.48, a carbon dioxide of 3.4 kilopascals, an oxygen level of 9.2 kilopascals, and a normal bicarbonate. Applied in sequence, the first question is the one that broke the working diagnosis. Her oxygen level was low despite a saturation of 96 percent and a respiratory rate of 32. A patient hyperventilating from anxiety alone should have an oxygen level at the upper end of normal, because they are moving a great deal of air through healthy lungs. Merritt was not oxygenating well despite substantial effort.

Intervention

The gas was escalated on the specific grounds that the oxygen level did not fit the working diagnosis. Imaging subsequently identified a pulmonary embolism. Anticoagulation was commenced.

Outcome

Merritt recovered and was discharged after five days. The case was reviewed locally. Notably, the two previous attendances had not included blood gas analysis, and the reviewers could not establish retrospectively whether the same process had been present on either occasion.

Teaching Points

A respiratory alkalosis with an unexpectedly low oxygen level is not a normal hyperventilation picture and warrants explanation.

Saturations of 96 percent excluded nothing. The oxygen level and the effort required to achieve it carried the diagnostic information.

A previous discharge with the same presentation is a reason for more scrutiny rather than less, though the opposite bias is well documented and was operating here.

3.7 Sampling and Reporting

A gas is only as good as the sample, and three handling errors account for most misleading results on a general ward.

Air bubbles in the syringe falsely raise the oxygen level and lower the carbon dioxide, because room air equilibrates with the sample. Expel bubbles immediately and cap the syringe. Delay before analysis allows ongoing cellular metabolism within the sample, which lowers the oxygen level and raises the carbon dioxide, so a sample analysed 20 minutes after collection may describe a patient who does not exist. Excess heparin dilutes the sample and shifts several values. None of these errors announce themselves on the printout.

Capillary earlobe sampling is a reasonable alternative in many ward situations and is considerably more comfortable for patients requiring repeated measurement. It gives a reliable carbon dioxide and pH. The oxygen value is less accurate than an arterial sample, which matters when oxygenation is the question and matters much less when the question is whether carbon dioxide is rising (O'Driscoll et al., 2017). For serial monitoring of a patient on ventilatory support, that trade off usually favours the earlobe.

Venous gases occupy a similar position. A venous sample will reliably exclude hypercapnia if the carbon dioxide is normal, which makes it a useful screening test. It cannot be used to grade the severity of established respiratory failure or to titrate ventilation.

Reporting is the final step and the one that determines whether any of this changes the patient's care. Two sentences work better than a recital of values. The first states the clinical situation and the second states the number that defines it. A nurse who says that a patient with COPD is more breathless than this morning and has a pH of 7.24 with a carbon dioxide of 9.1 has said everything required to generate an urgent review. A nurse who reads out 12 values in the order they appear on the printout has transferred the work of interpretation to somebody who is not standing at the bedside.

From Theory to Practice

Four questions, asked in the same order every time, will carry a ward nurse through the overwhelming majority of gases she will encounter. Oxygenation and the concentration it required. The pH and its severity. Whether carbon dioxide explains the pH. And what the bicarbonate says about how long this has been true.

The sequence is deliberately not a classification system. Naming a result correctly is a smaller achievement than knowing what to do with it, and the two skills come apart precisely in the cases where the stakes are highest. Merritt's gas would have been labelled respiratory alkalosis by any student with a mnemonic. What identified the embolism was the observation that one value did not belong with the others.

What this chapter cannot resolve is the decision that follows from a gas like Calloway's. Knowing that a patient has acute on chronic hypercapnic respiratory failure with a pH of 7.29 tells you the category. It does not tell you how long to persist with medical therapy before escalating, what pressures to expect, what the first hour should look like, or how to recognise the difference between a patient who is settling and a patient who is tiring while the numbers appear to improve. Those are the questions that determine whether the diagnosis you have just made changes anything, and they belong to Chapter 8.

Chapter 3 Review Questions

1. **A gas shows pH 7.36, carbon dioxide 7.9 kilopascals, bicarbonate 33 millimoles per litre, in a patient with known severe COPD who is comfortable at their usual baseline. What does this most likely represent?**

A) Acute hypercapnic respiratory failure requiring urgent ventilatory support

B) Chronic hypercapnia with established renal compensation

C) A metabolic alkalosis with respiratory compensation

D) A sampling error requiring an immediate repeat

Answer: B. The raised bicarbonate with a near normal pH indicates compensation developed over days or longer. The absolute carbon dioxide value is not the trigger for intervention. The pH is.

2. **Which value most reliably distinguishes acute deterioration from chronic hypercapnia?**

A) The absolute carbon dioxide level

B) The oxygen level

C) The pH

D) The oxygen saturation

Answer: C. Renal compensation cannot keep pace with an acute rise in carbon dioxide, so the pH falls. A patient may tolerate a markedly raised carbon dioxide for years with a near normal pH.

3. **Why does the sequence in this chapter begin with oxygenation rather than pH?**

A) Oxygenation is the most abnormal value in most gases

B) The oxygen level determines the acid base classification

C) Oxygenation and the concentration required to achieve it determine the most immediate nursing action

D) The pH is unreliable in samples analysed after a delay

Answer: C. The order is arranged by clinical urgency rather than by physiological logic. Classification can wait a further 20 seconds. Recognising that a normal oxygen level has been bought with 60 percent oxygen cannot.

PART II: OBSTRUCTIVE AIRWAY DISEASE

Chapter 4: Assessing COPD on Admission

Chapter Complexity Level: Intermediate

Prerequisites: Chapters 1 to 3.

Time Investment: One hour to read. One assessment to complete on shift.

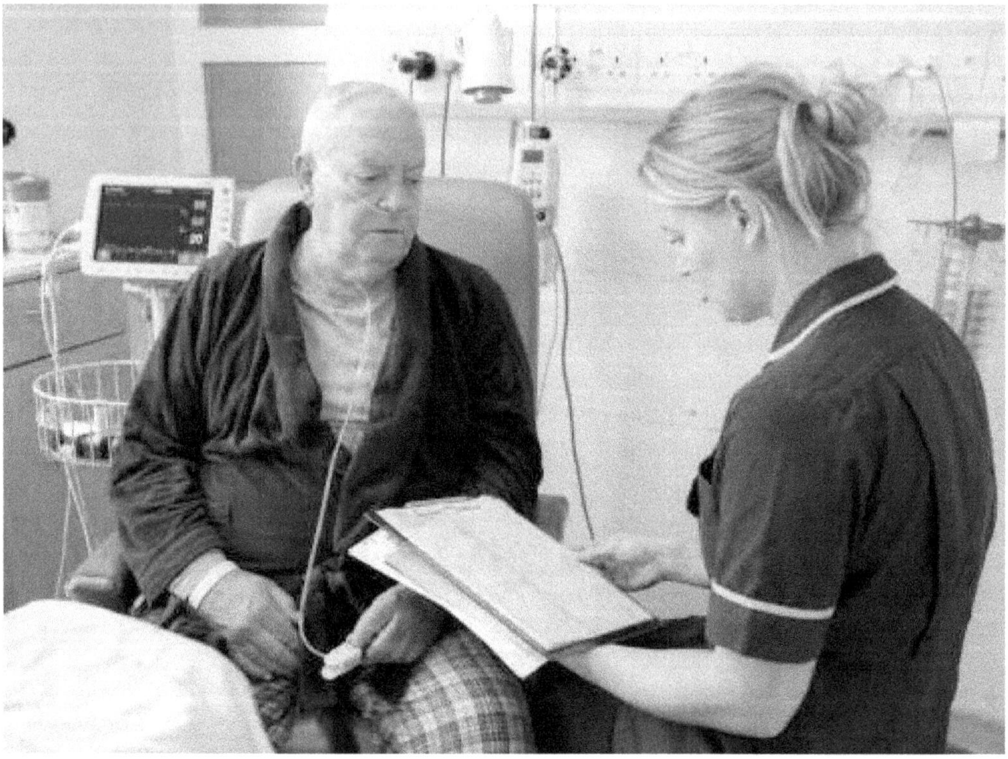

Lung function testing is the only way to confirm a diagnosis of chronic obstructive pulmonary disease. Lung function testing is also a poor predictor of which patients with that diagnosis will be admitted, readmitted, or die. Both statements are accurate, and they have been accurate for the entire working lifetime of most nurses reading this. The consequence is a condition that is defined by one measurement and managed according to another, which explains a good deal of the confusion that surrounds severity assessment on admission.

4.1 What Severity Actually Means

Ask three nurses how severe a patient's COPD is and you will get three different kinds of answer. One will quote a lung function percentage. One will describe how far the patient can walk. One will say that he is in every winter.

All three are describing something real, and they are describing different things. Airflow limitation, symptom burden, and exacerbation risk are separate axes. A patient can sit at an extreme of one and the middle of another. This is not a failure of the assessment tools. It is a property of the disease.

The practical implication for a nurse taking an admission is that severity cannot be captured in a single figure, and a handover that offers one has usually offered the least useful of the three.

4.2 From Lung Function to Risk

For most of the twentieth century, COPD severity meant airflow limitation, and airflow limitation meant the forced expiratory volume in one second expressed as a percentage of predicted. That measurement still defines the grades of airflow limitation, numbered one to four, and it still carries prognostic weight at the extremes.

Its limitations became difficult to ignore as outcome data accumulated. Patients with similar lung function had widely divergent symptoms and admission rates. Something other than the calibre of the airways was driving the difference.

The Global Initiative for Chronic Obstructive Lung Disease responded in 2011 with an assessment tool that combined symptoms and exacerbation history into four groups labelled A, B, C, and D. That tool was revised again in 2023. The two highest risk groups, C and D, were merged into a single group E, defined purely by exacerbation history and no longer subdivided by symptom burden (Global Initiative for Chronic Obstructive Lung Disease, 2025).

That merger is not a piece of administrative tidying. It encodes a clinical position, which is that a history of exacerbations predicts future risk so strongly that symptom level adds little once the exacerbation threshold has been crossed. A patient who exacerbates frequently is high risk whether or not they describe themselves as very breathless.

4.3 The ABE Framework

The current framework asks two questions and produces one of three groups.

The first question is about symptoms, assessed with a validated instrument rather than an impression. The second question is about exacerbations in the preceding 12 months, counting both those treated in the community and those requiring admission.

Group	Exacerbation history in past year	Symptom burden	What it signals
A	Zero or one, not requiring admission	Low	Lower risk, lower symptom burden
B	Zero or one, not requiring admission	High	Lower exacerbation risk, substantial daily impact
E	Two or more, or one requiring admission	Any level	High risk, regardless of symptom score

The single most important cell in that table is the one that appears twice in Group E. Symptom level does not modify the classification once the exacerbation criterion is met. A patient who describes only moderate breathlessness but who was admitted once in the past year sits in the highest risk group.

> **Teaching Point:** *Any patient you are admitting with an exacerbation has, by definition, met the criterion for Group E. The admission in front of you is itself the qualifying event, which means severity assessment is not something to complete at discharge planning. It is established on arrival.*

4.4 Measuring Symptoms Properly

Two instruments do the symptom work, and both take less time than the conversation nurses usually have instead.

The modified Medical Research Council dyspnoea scale grades breathlessness from zero to four by the activity that provokes it, ranging from breathlessness only on strenuous exercise to being too breathless to leave the house or breathless on dressing. It is quick, it is reproducible, and it measures one dimension only.

The COPD Assessment Test is an eight item questionnaire covering cough, sputum, chest tightness, breathlessness on exertion, activity limitation at home, confidence leaving the house, sleep, and energy. It produces a score from zero to 40. It captures the parts of the illness that a breathlessness scale misses entirely, and patients frequently score highly on items that nobody has ever asked them about.

The instruments have a use beyond classification. A patient who has never been asked about their confidence leaving the house is often surprised to find it is a legitimate clinical topic, and the answer opens a conversation about pulmonary rehabilitation that a breathlessness grade never would.

4.5 The Exacerbation Bundle

Assessment leads somewhere, and on admission it leads to a bundle of interventions delivered within the first few hours. The nursing contribution to that bundle is larger than the prescribing contribution, and it is the part most often delivered late.

Controlled oxygen comes first, targeted as described in Chapter 2. Bronchodilators follow, and the delivery decision here deserves attention. Nebulised bronchodilators are commonly used during an exacerbation, and in patients at risk of hypercapnia they should be driven by air rather than oxygen, with supplemental oxygen given by nasal cannulae alongside if required. A nebuliser driven by oxygen at 6 to 8 litres per minute delivers a high concentration continuously for the duration of the treatment, and a patient can accumulate carbon dioxide over three consecutive 20 minute nebulisers while everybody watches the saturations remain comfortable.

Systemic corticosteroids and antibiotics follow local protocol, with antibiotics indicated where sputum has become purulent (National Institute for Health and Care Excellence, 2019). The nursing tasks attached to these are unglamorous and consequential. Sputum should be sampled before antibiotics start rather than after. Blood glucose needs monitoring in patients receiving steroids, particularly those with existing diabetes, where a short course reliably destabilises control.

Venous thromboembolism assessment belongs in the first hours rather than the first ward round, because breathless immobile patients with an inflammatory illness sit squarely in the risk category, and because pulmonary embolism is among the conditions that mimic an exacerbation.

Early mobility is the element most often deferred and the one with the clearest downstream consequence. A patient who has not been out of bed by day two of an exacerbation is losing muscle at a rate that will affect their discharge date and their readmission risk. Sitting a breathless patient out for 20 minutes is a clinical intervention, not a comfort measure.

Smoking cessation is discussed in Chapter 16, because the timing of that conversation matters more than its content and the admission provides a specific window. What unites these elements is that none of them requires a decision from a prescriber, and all of them are routinely recorded as complete when they have in fact been deferred to the next shift.

4.6 What Gets Misunderstood

Three misunderstandings recur, and each one leads to a specific error.

The first is treating lung function as the master variable. A nurse who describes a patient as having mild COPD on the basis of preserved lung function, in a patient admitted for the third time in eight months, has described the airways accurately and the risk incorrectly.

The second is the assumption that severity assessment belongs to the specialist. It does not require specialist knowledge to ask eight questions and count admissions. It requires eight minutes.

The third is the most consequential. It is the assumption that a patient's presentation on admission reflects their baseline. It does not, and the entire concept of an exacerbation depends on the difference between the two. A patient who is breathless at rest may be at their normal state or may be in extremis, and the only way to know is to establish what they were like a week ago. That question is asked far less often than it should be, and it is the question section 4.7 turns on.

4.7 The Same Presentation, Different Baselines

The following are composite cases.

Case A

Oakley, aged 69, arrived by ambulance breathless at rest, saturations 87 percent on air, unable to complete a sentence. His wife reported that he had walked to the shop four days earlier and had been gardening the previous weekend. The change from baseline was dramatic. He was treated as a severe exacerbation, received prompt medical therapy and controlled oxygen, and improved substantially over 48 hours.

Case B

Fallon, aged 72, arrived the same afternoon breathless at rest, saturations 87 percent on air, unable to complete a sentence. She had not left her flat in seven months. She was breathless washing and dressing on a good day. Her presentation was almost identical to Oakley's and represented a far smaller change from her own baseline.

Fallon received the same treatment bundle, which was appropriate. What differed was what should have happened next. Oakley's admission was an acute event against a background of relative function. Fallon's was the visible part of a long decline, and the clinically significant finding in her case was not the saturation of 87 percent. It was that she had been housebound for seven months without anyone recording it, which placed her in Group E with a symptom burden that had never been measured and made her a candidate for a conversation about future care that had not yet happened.

The identical presentation carried entirely different information, and only the baseline distinguished them.

4.8 The Baseline Nobody Recorded

The following account is a composite, with details changed for anonymity.

Briar was a Band 6 on an acute medical unit and had developed a habit that her colleagues found mildly irritating. On every COPD admission she asked the same question before anything else, which was what the patient had been able to do a week ago.

On one admission the answer was that the patient had been managing the stairs to his flat, slowly, with two rests. He was now unable to move from the chair to the commode. Nothing in the observations distinguished him from the four other COPD patients on the unit that evening. His saturations were 90 percent, his respiratory rate was 24, and his early warning score was unremarkable.

Briar escalated on the basis of the change and was initially told that his observations did not support urgent review. She persisted, and the phrase she used was that he had lost two flights of stairs in seven days. He was reviewed, found to have a pH of 7.30 with a raised carbon dioxide, and commenced on noninvasive ventilation that evening.

The uncomfortable part of this account is what happened three weeks later, when a similar patient was admitted to the same unit while Briar was on nights elsewhere. The baseline question was not asked. The patient was reviewed at the routine time, six hours after admission, and by then required a higher level of intervention. No harm was formally attributed. The unit did not change its documentation, and as far as the author is aware, the question is still asked by some nurses and not by others, which is the ordinary fate of most good practice that depends on individuals rather than systems.

Teaching points:

Functional change over days is a more sensitive marker of exacerbation severity than any single observation, and it is not recorded on any standard chart.

A practice that depends entirely on one nurse's habit is not a practice. It is a personal standard, and it leaves with her at the end of the shift.

What Holds Up

Three things survive scrutiny. Exacerbation history predicts future exacerbations more reliably than lung function does, which is why the 2023 revision collapsed two groups into one on that basis alone. Symptom burden and airflow limitation measure genuinely different things and neither substitutes for the other. And functional change from baseline, which appears in no classification system at all, carries more information about the severity of the episode in front of you than the classification does.

What remains contested is what to do with that last point. The measurement instruments in section 4.4 are validated, reproducible, and designed for stable disease assessed in clinic. The baseline question in section 4.8 is none of those things. It is unvalidated, it depends on recall, it is frequently answered by a relative rather than the patient, and it does not appear on an admission proforma anywhere the author has worked.

It is also, in the specific setting of an acute admission, the more useful question. That is an uncomfortable position to hold, and it should be held with appropriate hesitancy. The honest summary is that the validated tools tell you where a patient sits in a population, and the unvalidated question tells you what has changed in this person this week. Assessment on admission needs both, and only one of them has a box on the form.

Chapter 4 Review Questions

1. **A patient with COPD has a low symptom score and was admitted once in the past 12 months with an exacerbation. Which group does the current GOLD framework place them in?**

A) Group A, because symptom burden is low

B) Group B, because they have had one exacerbation

C) Group E, because an exacerbation requiring admission meets the criterion regardless of symptoms

D) The group cannot be determined without lung function results

Answer: C. Since the 2023 revision, a single exacerbation requiring hospitalisation places a patient in Group E irrespective of symptom level. Lung function grades airflow limitation separately and does not determine the group.

2. **Which assessment provides the most information about the severity of the acute episode in front of you?**

A) The percentage predicted forced expiratory volume in one second

B) The change in functional capacity over the preceding days

C) The oxygen saturation on arrival

D) The number of inhalers on the prescription

Answer: B. Change from baseline defines an exacerbation. A saturation of 87 percent may be normal or catastrophic for a given patient, as the paired cases in section 4.7 illustrate.

3. **What is the principal limitation of the modified Medical Research Council dyspnoea scale as a sole symptom measure?**

A) It requires spirometry to interpret

B) It measures breathlessness only and misses cough, sputum, sleep, and confidence

C) It cannot be used in patients over 70

D) It is not validated in COPD

Answer: B. It is a single dimension instrument. The COPD Assessment Test covers the additional domains and frequently identifies problems that have never been raised.

Chapter 5: Inhalers and the Competence Gap

Chapter Complexity Level: Intermediate

Prerequisites: Chapter 4. Access to the inhaler devices stocked on your unit.

Time Investment: One hour to read. Twenty minutes to self assess before reading section 5.3.

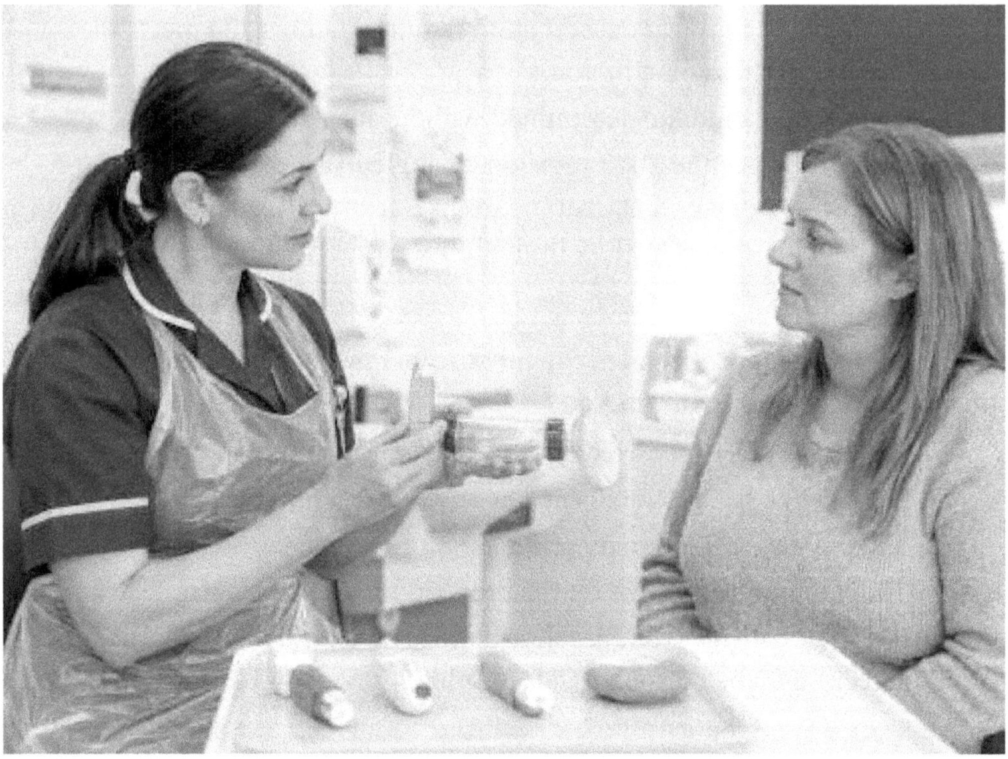

The nurses least likely to teach inhaler technique correctly are not the inexperienced ones. In a specialised respiratory inpatient unit, researchers assessed 25 nurses on their competence with eight inhaler devices and separately on their confidence in delivering inhaler education. Eighty four percent described themselves as moderately or extremely confident. The mean proportion of correct steps was 47 percent. Confidence had no relationship with competence, and neither did years of nursing experience (Swami et al., 2021). Something else predicted competence, and what it was matters for how this chapter is organised.

5.1 The Problem Nobody Measures

Inhaled therapy is the foundation of treatment for both major obstructive airway diseases. A drug delivered by an incorrectly used device does not reach the lungs, which means an inhaler technique error is a total treatment failure that looks identical to treatment resistance.

The patient is not the only variable. The chain runs from prescriber to device to teaching to patient performance, and the teaching link is the one nobody measures. Inhaler technique in patients is audited routinely in some services. Inhaler technique in the staff teaching them is audited almost nowhere.

The consequence is a specific and slightly humiliating pattern. A patient's technique is checked, found to be poor, corrected by a nurse whose own technique is imperfect, and documented as taught. The documentation is accurate. The teaching was delivered. What was taught was partially wrong.

Before reading further, do this. Take each device stocked on your unit, without a placebo trainer if none is available, and write down every step in order for each one. Then compare against section 5.3. Most readers will score somewhere between 40 and 60 percent, which is unpleasant and is precisely the result the research predicts.

5.2 Why Training Has Not Fixed It

Inhaler technique education has been delivered to nursing staff for decades. The persistence of the problem despite that effort suggests the training design is at fault rather than the effort.

Three features explain most of it. Training is usually delivered once, at induction or on a study day, and technique decays measurably within weeks without reinforcement. Training usually covers the devices the trainer knows rather than the devices the ward stocks, and formularies change faster than teaching materials. And training is almost always assessed by attendance rather than by demonstration, which means a nurse can complete inhaler training and never once have been watched using an inhaler.

The Swami study found one variable that did predict competence, and it was not seniority or confidence. It was the number of prescriptions for that specific device issued in the hospital in the preceding year. Nurses were good at the devices they saw constantly and poor at the rest. That finding points directly at the design of any remedy. Competence follows exposure, so any teaching that is not organised around the devices actually in use on your unit will decay in the same way its predecessors did.

5.3 Critical Errors by Device Class

Not all errors matter equally. A **critical error** is one that substantially or completely prevents drug reaching the lower airways. Distinguishing critical from minor errors is what allows a nurse to correct the two things that matter in a 90 second interaction rather than reciting 11 steps that a breathless patient will not retain.

Device class	Inhalation manoeuvre	The critical errors
Pressurised metered dose inhaler	Slow and deep, actuate at the start of inhalation	Failure to coordinate actuation with inhalation. Failure to shake. No breath hold. Inhaling too fast
Metered dose inhaler with spacer	Slow and deep, or tidal breathing	Delay of more than a few seconds between actuation and inhalation. Multiple doses fired into the chamber at once
Dry powder inhaler	Quick and deep, forceful from the start	Inhaling slowly. Exhaling into the device. Failure to load or pierce the dose. Holding the device incorrectly during loading
Breath actuated inhaler	Steady and deep until the device fires	Stopping inhalation when the device clicks. Failure to prime or open the cap fully
Soft mist inhaler	Slow and deep, actuate at the start	Failure to prime a new device. Inhaling too fast. Not turning the base fully before use

Two errors on that table are worth isolating because they account for a disproportionate share of failures and because they are opposites.

A pressurised metered dose inhaler requires a slow inhalation, because the aerosol is already travelling fast and rapid inhalation drives it into the back of the throat. A dry powder inhaler requires a fast inhalation, because the patient's own inspiratory flow is what disaggregates the powder. Teaching a patient slow and deep for every device, which is the commonest error made by staff, disables every dry powder inhaler they own.

The second is the breath hold. Ten seconds where possible, or as long as is comfortable, allows aerosol deposition rather than immediate exhalation. It is omitted more often than any other step and it is the easiest to reinstate.

> **Teaching Point:** *If you correct only two things in a patient's technique, correct the inhalation speed for the device class and reinstate the breath hold. Those two changes recover more delivered drug than any other pair of corrections available to you.*

5.4 Spacers

Spacers solve the coordination problem, reduce oropharyngeal deposition, and are useful across a far wider population than the paediatric and elderly groups they are often reserved for.

Three practical points determine whether a spacer works. New plastic spacers carry an electrostatic charge that attracts drug particles to the chamber wall, which is why priming with several actuations or washing in detergent and allowing to air dry without rinsing is recommended. Rinsing and drying with a cloth restores the charge, which makes the well intentioned act of towel drying a spacer counterproductive.

Actuate one dose at a time. Firing two or three doses into the chamber before inhaling reduces delivery rather than increasing it, because the particles collide and deposit.

And inhale promptly. Aerosol in a chamber settles within seconds, so a delay between actuation and inhalation loses drug rapidly. Tidal breathing through the chamber for five breaths works as well as a single slow deep breath in most patients and is easier for a breathless one.

5.5 Teaching Without Patronising

The following account is a composite, with details changed for anonymity.

Joss had been checking inhaler technique on a respiratory ward for two years and had developed a reliable way of making patients defensive. He would ask whether they knew how to use their inhaler. Everybody said yes. He would then watch them do it wrong and correct them, and a proportion of patients would explain that they had been using it that way for 20 years and that no doctor had ever complained.

The change he made was small and it was to the opening. Instead of asking whether the patient knew how to use the device, he began saying that the devices are genuinely awkward, that most people have at least one step slightly off, and that he would like to watch so he could see which one it was for them. Almost nobody refused, and almost nobody became defensive, because the framing located the problem in the device rather than in the patient.

The step that took longer to learn was to stop talking during the demonstration. His instinct had been to coach as the patient inhaled, which meant he was correcting an error he had partly caused by interrupting. Watching in silence, then correcting once, produced a more accurate picture of what the patient did at home.

Not everything improved. A proportion of patients with long established technique reverted within weeks, and Joss's unit had no mechanism for rechecking after discharge. The section 5.2 finding that competence follows exposure applies to patients as directly as it does to staff, and a single teaching episode on an acute ward is a weak intervention against 20 years of habit.

Teaching points:

Locating the difficulty in the device rather than the person removes most of the defensiveness that makes technique checks unproductive.

Watching in silence before correcting produces a more accurate assessment than coaching in real time.

5.6 The Treatment That Never Arrived

The following is a composite case; identifying details have been changed.

Background

Linden, aged 63, had a diagnosis of COPD made six years earlier and had been admitted four times in 18 months with exacerbations. Her maintenance therapy had been escalated twice, most recently to a combination inhaler delivered by dry powder device.

Presentation

She presented with her fourth exacerbation, describing no benefit whatsoever from the most recent change in therapy. Her symptom score was high, her exercise tolerance had declined steadily, and the working assumption documented in her notes was that her disease was progressing and that further escalation should be considered.

Analysis

On the second day of admission a nurse asked her to demonstrate her inhaler. She loaded the device correctly, exhaled into the mouthpiece, and then inhaled slowly and gently over about four seconds. Exhaling into a dry powder device disperses the loaded dose and introduces moisture. Inhaling slowly fails to disaggregate whatever powder remains. She had almost certainly received minimal drug from that device since it was prescribed, and the same manoeuvre would have partly disabled the previous one.

Intervention

Technique was corrected and she was switched to a device requiring a different manoeuvre after discussion with the respiratory team, on the grounds that her established habit was slow inhalation and that fighting it was less reliable than accommodating it. She was taught with a placebo device and asked to demonstrate back on three separate occasions before discharge.

Outcome

At six weeks her symptom score had improved and she had not required rescue treatment. She had not, however, returned to her previous exercise tolerance, and it is not possible to say retrospectively how much irreversible decline occurred during the period when her maintenance therapy was not being delivered. Two of her four admissions had been attributed to disease progression.

Teaching Points

Apparent treatment failure should prompt a technique check before it prompts an escalation in therapy.

Matching the device to the patient's existing manoeuvre is often more reliable than retraining the manoeuvre, particularly where the habit is long established.

Documented technique teaching and verified technique are different things, and only the second requires the patient to demonstrate.

5.7 Matching Device to Patient

Linden's case turned on a decision that nurses influence more than they realise, which is which device a patient is given in the first place.

Inspiratory flow is the deciding variable. Dry powder devices require the patient to generate sufficient flow to disaggregate the powder, and that requirement differs between devices because internal resistance differs. A patient with severe airflow limitation, significant frailty, or an acute exacerbation may be unable to generate adequate flow through a higher resistance device, and the same patient may manage perfectly well when stable. Prescribing a dry powder device during an exacerbation, on the evidence of a demonstration given while the patient is unwell, is a decision worth revisiting before discharge.

Pressurised metered dose inhalers make the opposite demand. They require no inspiratory effort but they require coordination, which is the capacity most affected by cognitive impairment, arthritis in the hands, and acute breathlessness. A spacer removes the coordination requirement entirely, which is why the combination of a pressurised inhaler and a spacer is frequently the most reliable option for the patients whose technique is hardest to correct.

Three practical questions settle most device decisions at the bedside. Can the patient generate a forceful inhalation. Can they coordinate hand and breath. Can they physically manipulate the device, including opening a cap, twisting a base, or piercing a capsule, with the hands they have on a bad day.

That last question is asked least and answered most decisively. A patient with rheumatoid changes in the hands may understand every step and be unable to load the device. No amount of teaching corrects a mechanical problem, and it is the kind of finding that becomes obvious in ten seconds of watching and remains invisible across years of asking.

Device choice also carries an environmental dimension that patients increasingly raise. Propellant based inhalers have a substantially higher carbon footprint than dry powder devices. That is a legitimate consideration in a shared decision, and it is not a reason to place a patient on a device they cannot generate sufficient flow to use.

Closing the Loop

Linden's notes recorded that inhaler technique had been checked on two previous admissions. Both entries were truthful. Somebody had asked her whether she knew how to use her inhaler, she had said yes, and the box had been completed. What had never happened, across four admissions and six years, was that anybody watched her do it.

That gap between checked and watched is the whole subject of this chapter, and it exists on both sides of the interaction. Staff who have never been observed using the devices teach patients who are never observed using them, and the documentation records that education has taken place. The Swami finding that confidence predicted nothing is uncomfortable precisely because confidence is what fills that gap when observation is absent.

The remedy is unglamorous. Assess yourself against the critical errors in section 5.3 before you teach. Correct the inhalation speed and the breath hold in preference to anything else. Watch in silence, then correct once. Ask for a demonstration back, on more than one occasion, and record what the patient actually did rather than that teaching was given.

None of that requires a study day, a competency framework, or permission. It requires accepting, once, that the 47 percent figure probably describes you, which is the least comfortable and most useful assumption available in this chapter.

Chapter 5 Review Questions

1. **A patient using a dry powder inhaler inhales slowly and gently over four seconds. Why is this a critical error?**

A) It causes excessive oropharyngeal deposition of the drug

B) The patient's inspiratory flow is required to disaggregate the powder, and slow inhalation fails to do this

C) It prevents the device from loading the next dose

D) It shortens the effective breath hold

Answer: B. Dry powder devices are passive and rely entirely on the patient's inspiratory effort. The correct manoeuvre is quick and deep, which is the opposite of that required for a pressurised metered dose inhaler.

2. **A patient fires three doses into a spacer before inhaling, in order to save time. What is the effect?**

A) Delivery is increased proportionally

B) Delivery is unchanged

C) Delivery is reduced, because particles collide and deposit within the chamber

D) Delivery is unaffected but the spacer requires immediate cleaning

Answer: C. Each dose should be actuated separately and inhaled promptly. Multiple actuations reduce the drug available for inhalation.

3. **A patient reports no benefit from a recently escalated maintenance inhaler. What should be considered before further escalation?**

A) A trial of oral therapy

B) Verified inhaler technique, demonstrated by the patient rather than reported

C) Repeat lung function testing

D) An increase in the prescribed dose

Answer: B. Apparent treatment failure caused by technique error is indistinguishable from disease progression on history alone, and escalating therapy delivered by a device the patient cannot use does not correct the underlying problem.

Chapter 6: Asthma After the Guideline Change

Chapter Complexity Level: Intermediate

Prerequisites: Chapter 5. Familiarity with the inhaled therapies stocked locally.

Time Investment: One hour to read. One drug chart review to complete.

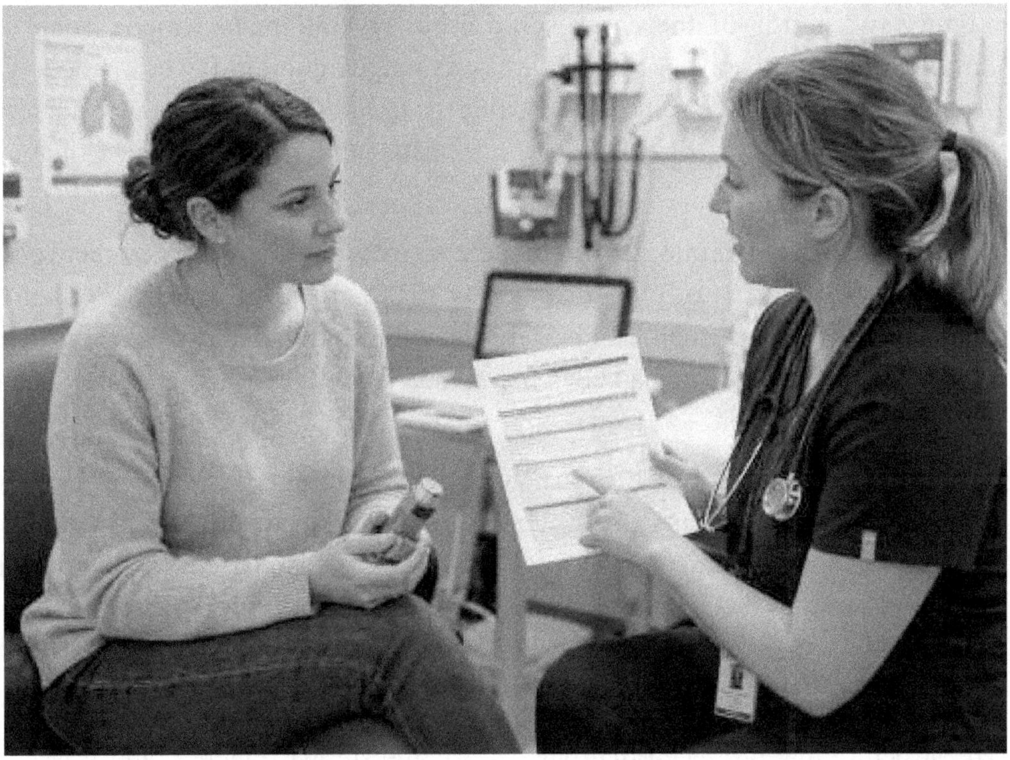

In November 2024, the British Thoracic Society, the National Institute for Health and Care Excellence, and the Scottish Intercollegiate Guidelines Network published a single joint asthma guideline, replacing two separate documents that had guided United Kingdom practice for years. Buried in the pharmacological section was a sentence that reversed something almost every nurse in the country had been taught. For people aged 12 and over, short acting reliever therapy used alone was no longer recommended, and combination inhaled corticosteroid with formoterol, used either as needed or as maintenance and reliever therapy, became the foundation of treatment (British Thoracic Society, National Institute for Health and Care Excellence, & Scottish Intercollegiate Guidelines Network, 2024). The blue inhaler had been the universal symbol of asthma for four decades. It had also been implicated in deaths for nearly as long.

6.1 The Problem Before the Change

The case for change was built on death certificates rather than on trial data alone.

The National Review of Asthma Deaths examined 276 sets of records of people certified as having died from asthma in the United Kingdom over a 12 month period from February 2012. It found potentially preventable factors in roughly two thirds of the cases scrutinised. Overall management, acute and chronic, in primary and secondary care, was judged good in fewer than one fifth of those who died. Assessors identified a failure by doctors and nurses to recognise and act on risk factors for attacks and death (Royal College of Physicians, 2014).

Two prescribing findings from that enquiry did more to change practice than any other single piece of evidence. Thirty nine percent of those who died had been prescribed more than 12 short acting reliever inhalers in the year before death. Thirty eight percent had been prescribed fewer than four preventer inhalers in the same period.

Those two numbers describe a treatment pattern rather than a treatment failure. Patients were being given increasing quantities of the drug that relieved symptoms and insufficient quantities of the drug that treated the underlying inflammation, and the relief was masking the deterioration.

6.2 The Ladder That Shaped a Generation

The structure that produced that pattern was the stepwise ladder, and it is worth understanding because most patients currently on a ward were started on it.

The ladder began with a reliever alone for mild intermittent asthma. A preventer was added if the reliever was needed frequently. Further agents were added at higher steps. The logic was proportionate and intuitive, and it embedded an assumption that turned out to be wrong, which was that mild asthma is primarily a symptom problem and only becomes an inflammatory problem when symptoms become frequent.

Two consequences followed from that assumption. Patients spent time on reliever only treatment with untreated airway inflammation. And the reliever, being the drug that produced immediate perceptible benefit, acquired a psychological primacy that the preventer never achieved. Patients carried the blue inhaler. They kept the brown one in a cupboard.

The ladder also created a monitoring problem. Reliever use is a marker of disease control, but under a stepwise system it was also a legitimate treatment at the lowest step, which made high reliever use ambiguous. It could mean uncontrolled disease or it could mean mild disease being managed as designed.

6.3 What the Evidence Overturned

The pivot came from trials of as needed combination inhaled corticosteroid with formoterol against as needed reliever alone in mild asthma.

Formoterol is the component that made the strategy possible. It is a long acting bronchodilator with a rapid onset, which means a single inhaler can serve as both reliever and preventer. Every time the patient treats a symptom, they also deliver a dose of anti inflammatory treatment. The behaviour that previously masked deterioration now treats it.

The trial evidence showed substantial reductions in severe exacerbations compared with as needed reliever alone, and outcomes comparable to or better than regular low dose preventer plus as needed reliever, despite considerably lower total steroid exposure. Adherence explains part of that result. Patients take treatment when they feel symptoms, reliably, and take daily preventive treatment when they feel well far less reliably.

The Medicines and Healthcare products Regulatory Agency reinforced the position in April 2025 with a reminder about the risks of reliever overuse in asthma and the changes to prescribing guidance that had followed (Medicines and Healthcare products Regulatory Agency, 2025).

> **Teaching Point:** *Under the current framework, a patient collecting large numbers of reliever inhalers is not simply poorly controlled. They are on a regimen that current guidance no longer recommends, and the finding belongs in a message to a prescriber rather than in a note about adherence.*

6.4 AIR and MART in Practice

Two regimens follow from the change, and nurses need to distinguish them because patients confuse them constantly.

Anti inflammatory reliever therapy, abbreviated to AIR, means a low dose combination inhaler taken only when symptoms occur. There is no scheduled daily dose. It replaces reliever only treatment for patients at the mild end.

Maintenance and reliever therapy, abbreviated to MART, means the same combination inhaler taken on a fixed schedule every day and additionally when symptoms occur. One inhaler, two purposes, and a maximum number of daily doses that the patient must know.

Four counselling points determine whether either regimen works, and all four are nursing tasks.

The patient must understand that there is no separate rescue inhaler. This is the point patients find hardest, and many keep an old reliever in a bag for reassurance. That retained inhaler is not neutral. It allows the patient to treat symptoms without delivering the anti inflammatory component, which reconstructs the exact problem the strategy was designed to solve.

The patient must know their maximum daily doses and what to do on reaching it, which is to seek urgent review rather than to continue.

The patient must understand that increased use during a deterioration is the intended behaviour rather than a sign of failure. Under the old ladder, needing more reliever meant treatment was inadequate. Under MART, needing more of the combination inhaler is the treatment.

Where control is not achieved despite escalation through moderate dose maintenance and reliever therapy and trials of additional agents, referral to a specialist asthma service is recommended (British Thoracic Society et al., 2025).

And the patient must have a written personal asthma action plan. The enquiry that drove all of this identified failure to provide action plans as a recurring preventable factor. An action plan that lives in a discharge letter is not an action plan. It has to be in the patient's possession, written in the number of doses their actual inhaler delivers, and specific about the point at which they stop self managing and seek help. Plans written generically, without the patient's own device and doses on them, are among the commonest documentation artefacts on a respiratory ward and among the least used at home.

6.5 Two Patients, One Change

The following are composite cases.

Case A

Arden, aged 34, was switched from a reliever plus separate preventer to a MART regimen during an outpatient review. The nurse who made the change spent 12 minutes on it. She had Arden state back the maximum daily doses, asked what he would do if he reached it, and asked him to bring in every inhaler he had at home at the next appointment. He brought four, two of which were expired relievers. They were disposed of together. Over the following year he had one course of oral steroids, down from three the year before.

Case B

Vesper, aged 31, was switched to the same regimen on discharge from an emergency department attendance. She was handed the new inhaler with a leaflet. She continued using her old reliever for symptoms, because that was what a reliever was for, and used the new inhaler twice daily as she understood the instruction. Her total anti inflammatory dose was therefore fixed, her symptom driven doses delivered no steroid, and she re presented within four months.

The prescription was identical in both cases. What differed was whether anyone established what the patient would do with the old inhaler, which takes under a minute to ask and is the single question that separates a working MART regimen from a broken one.

6.6 The Patient Nobody Reviewed

The following account is a composite, with details changed for anonymity.

Pax had been a practice nurse for 11 years and ran the asthma reviews at her surgery. She had been trained on the stepwise ladder, had taught it to students, and had been broadly aware that a new guideline had been published without having examined what it required of her.

The prompt to look was a search she ran for a different purpose. Reviewing patients overdue an annual check, she noticed how many were on reliever only treatment. When she counted, it came to a substantial proportion of her asthma register, most of them young adults who never attended, several with prescription records showing repeated reliever collection and no preventer collection at all.

Her first instinct was to book them all in, and it failed. The patients who do not attend annual reviews are, definitionally, the patients who do not attend when invited. Attendance for her first round of invitations was under a third.

What worked better was to change the trigger. She arranged for reliever prescription requests above a threshold to generate a prompt at the point of the request rather than a letter, on the reasoning that a patient asking for an inhaler wants something and is therefore reachable in a way that a patient receiving a letter is not.

It is worth being honest about the limits of what she achieved. She reached more patients than before, not all of them. The enquiry recommendations she was implementing were published in 2014, and she was implementing them a decade later, which is a reasonable description of how guideline change usually propagates into routine practice.

Teaching points:

Prescription collection records identify at risk patients more reliably than symptom reports, because they capture behaviour rather than recall.

The patients most at risk are the least likely to attend a review, so an intervention that depends on attendance will systematically miss them.

6.7 The Diagnosis Nobody Confirmed

The 2024 guideline made a second change that received far less attention than the treatment reversal and that has equally direct consequences on a ward.

Asthma now requires objective confirmation. A suggestive history is the starting point rather than the diagnosis, and it must be supported by testing. Fractional exhaled nitric oxide, which measures a marker of eosinophilic airway inflammation, has a defined place. So does spirometry with bronchodilator reversibility, blood eosinophil measurement, and peak flow variability recorded over a period.

The reason this matters clinically is contained in one of the more startling findings of the National Review of Asthma Deaths. A substantial proportion of the people whose records were examined turned out not to have died from asthma at all, and in a considerable number of cases the records contained no evident rationale for the asthma diagnosis in the first place (Royal College of Physicians, 2014).

A diagnosis attached to a patient in childhood, never revisited, generates two distinct harms. It exposes people without asthma to long term inhaled therapy and to the assumption that any breathlessness they develop is asthma, which delays the identification of heart failure, obesity related breathlessness, and dysfunctional breathing. And it removes the diagnostic scrutiny from patients who do have asthma but whose deterioration gets attributed to a label rather than investigated.

The nursing contribution here is narrower than the prescribing contribution but it is not negligible. Peak flow diaries are nurse initiated in most services, and a patient who leaves an admission with a meter, a chart, and an understanding of what twice daily readings are for supplies data that no single clinic measurement can. Asking a patient with a decades old asthma label what testing was originally done is a reasonable question, and the answer is frequently that nobody knows. That answer is worth recording in the notes rather than letting it pass, because an unexamined label survives indefinitely until somebody writes down that it has never been examined.

Looking Back and Ahead

The enquiry that identified excessive reliever prescribing as a preventable factor in asthma deaths reported in 2014. The guideline that removed reliever only treatment from the recommended pathway was published in 2024. Ten years separated the finding from the structural response, and the finding itself restated a pattern that had been identified in studies of asthma deaths for over half a century.

That interval is the uncomfortable part of this chapter. The evidence about reliever overuse was not obscure, contested, or newly discovered. It was known, published, and widely cited throughout the period in which prescribing continued substantially as before.

Which raises the question this chapter leaves the reader holding. Every nurse reading this can now identify a patient on an outdated regimen, because the criteria are simple and the prescription record is visible. The knowledge is no longer the barrier. So what is it that stands between recognising such a patient on a drug chart on a Tuesday afternoon and something changing for them, and how much of that distance is made up of things a nurse at the bedside can actually close?

Some of it is prescribing authority, which most readers do not hold. Rather less of it than is usually assumed. Vesper's regimen failed for want of a question about an old inhaler, and that question requires no authority whatsoever.

Chapter 6 Review Questions

1. **Under the 2024 joint asthma guideline, what is recommended for a patient aged over 12 with confirmed asthma currently using a short acting reliever alone?**

A) Continue the reliever and add a separate daily preventer

B) Change to a low dose combination inhaled corticosteroid with formoterol used as needed

C) Continue unchanged if symptoms occur less than twice weekly

D) Refer directly to a specialist asthma service

Answer: B. Reliever only treatment is no longer recommended in this age group. Anti inflammatory reliever therapy is the recommended replacement, with maintenance and reliever therapy used where control requires it.

2. **A patient on a MART regimen also keeps an old short acting reliever inhaler and uses it for symptoms. Why does this undermine the regimen?**

A) The two drugs interact and reduce bronchodilation

B) Symptom driven doses no longer deliver the anti inflammatory component

C) The patient will exceed the maximum daily dose of formoterol

D) It invalidates the personal asthma action plan

Answer: B. The mechanism of MART depends on every symptom driven dose also delivering inhaled corticosteroid. A retained reliever restores the original problem of symptom relief without inflammatory treatment.

3. **Which prescribing pattern was identified as a preventable factor in the National Review of Asthma Deaths?**

A) Prescription of long acting bronchodilators without specialist review

B) High reliever prescription volume combined with low preventer prescription volume

C) Prescription of oral corticosteroids for more than five days

D) Use of spacers in adults

Answer: B. The enquiry found that 39 percent of those who died had received more than 12 reliever inhalers in the preceding year and 38 percent fewer than four preventer inhalers.

Chapter 7: Acute Severe Asthma

Chapter Complexity Level: Advanced

Prerequisites: Chapters 1, 2, and 6.

Time Investment: One hour to read. Six grading vignettes to work through.

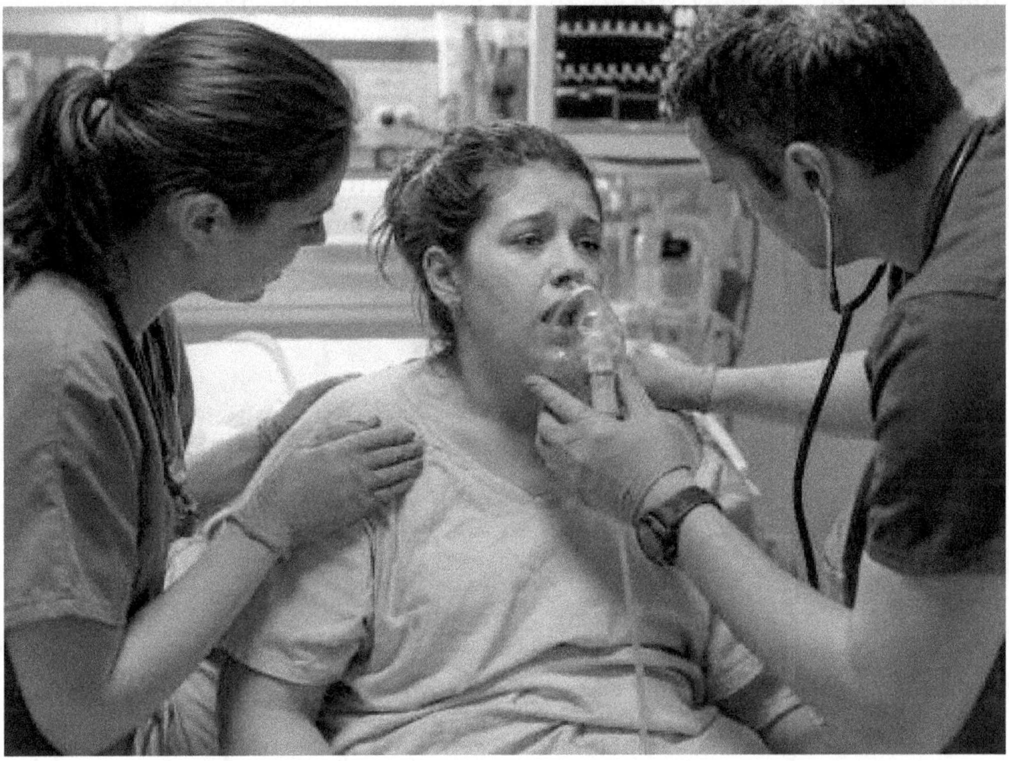

The wheeze had been audible from the corridor at ten past three. At twenty five past, standing at the same bed space, the nurse could not hear it any more. The patient was sitting upright, both hands gripping the mattress, and had not spoken since the second nebuliser. Her chest moved. Air did not appear to be moving with it. The registrar, arriving from another ward, said that she sounded better. He was describing what he could hear, which was almost nothing, and he was describing it as improvement. The next four minutes determined the outcome of the admission, and nothing that happened in them was written in a protocol.

7.1 What Was Happening

Kestrel was 24 and had been admitted three hours earlier with an asthma attack that had begun the previous evening. She had used her reliever inhaler repeatedly through the night. She had not sought help until her partner insisted in the morning.

On arrival she had a respiratory rate of 30, a heart rate of 128, saturations of 91 percent on air, and a peak flow she was unable to perform adequately. She received oxygen, nebulised bronchodilators, and oral corticosteroids. Over the following two hours her wheeze diminished, her respiratory rate fell from 30 to 24, and her heart rate came down slightly. The observation chart recorded a gradual improvement, and by any reading of the numbers alone it was a patient responding to treatment.

The nurse who noticed at twenty five past three had been in the bay for the whole period. What alarmed her was not any single measurement. It was that Kestrel had stopped talking, that her respiratory effort had increased while her respiratory rate had fallen, and that the chest had become quiet without the patient becoming comfortable.

She escalated as a life threatening attack. Kestrel was moved to the high dependency area, received intravenous magnesium and continuous nebulisation, and did not require intubation. She was discharged after six days.

7.2 Why the Numbers Improved

The reassuring trajectory on Kestrel's chart was real, and it was measuring the wrong thing.

Wheeze is generated by turbulent airflow through narrowed airways. It requires airflow. As bronchoconstriction becomes extreme, or as the patient tires and generates less flow, the wheeze diminishes and eventually disappears. The **silent chest** is therefore not the resolution of wheeze. It is the loss of the airflow that was producing it, and it is one of the features that defines a life threatening attack.

The falling respiratory rate followed the same logic. A rate of 30 in a patient fighting hard is a compensating patient. A rate of 24 in a patient who has been fighting for 18 hours may be a patient who can no longer sustain 30. Chapter 1 established that a falling respiratory rate is improvement in a patient who is brightening and a terminal sign in a patient who is tiring, and asthma is where that distinction is made most often and most urgently.

The heart rate did not fall much, and this is the value that fits least comfortably into a reassuring narrative. Persistent tachycardia in a patient whose respiratory rate is falling deserves explanation, and exhaustion explains it better than recovery does.

> **Teaching Point:** *In acute asthma, treat a quiet chest as an emergency finding until proven otherwise. The absence of wheeze in a distressed patient is not the absence of bronchospasm. It is the absence of air movement.*

7.3 Grading the Attack

Attacks are graded because the grade determines the setting, the monitoring interval, and the escalation threshold. The categories below reflect long standing United Kingdom practice, incorporated into the acute asthma section of the current pathway (British Thoracic Society et al., 2024).

Grade	Defining features	What it means operationally
Moderate	Increasing symptoms, peak flow above 50 percent of best or predicted, no features of severe asthma	Treat and reassess. Usually manageable in a standard ward area
Acute severe	Peak flow 33 to 50 percent, respiratory rate 25 or more, heart rate 110 or more, or inability to complete sentences in one breath	Any single feature qualifies. Requires close monitoring and senior review
Life threatening	Silent chest, poor respiratory effort, cyanosis, exhaustion, altered consciousness, arrhythmia, hypotension, saturations below 92 percent, peak flow below 33 percent	Immediate critical care involvement. Blood gas required
Near fatal	Raised carbon dioxide, or requirement for mechanical ventilation	Carbon dioxide should be low in acute asthma. A normal or raised value is an emergency finding

Two points about this table cause more confusion than the rest combined.

Any single feature places the patient in that grade. A patient who can talk normally, looks comfortable, and has a heart rate of 112 has acute severe asthma by definition. The instinct to average the features and arrive at a moderate impression is the commonest grading error.

And the carbon dioxide criterion runs opposite to intuition. In acute asthma, patients hyperventilate, so carbon dioxide should be low. A normal carbon dioxide in an acutely asthmatic patient means ventilation has fallen to the point where the compensation has been lost, and it belongs in the near fatal category rather than in the reassuring one. This is the exact reverse of the interpretation applied to COPD in Chapter 3, and the two must not be confused.

7.4 Nursing Actions in Sequence

The interventions themselves are prescribed. The sequencing, monitoring, and escalation are nursing work.

Oxygen comes first, targeted at 94 to 98 percent. Acute asthma is not a hypercapnia risk group in the sense described in Chapter 2, and the lower target range does not apply unless the patient has a separate documented reason for it.

Bronchodilators follow, nebulised and oxygen driven in this population, repeated or given continuously according to severity and response. Corticosteroids should be given early, and the interval between arrival and administration is a reasonable local audit measure because it is frequently longer than anyone believes.

Magnesium and intravenous therapies belong to the severe and life threatening categories and are prescribed decisions. The nursing task attached to them is preparation and monitoring, and specifically the recognition that a patient requiring them has already crossed into a category needing critical care input.

Monitoring intervals matter as much as the drugs. A patient with acute severe asthma needs continuous oximetry and observations at intervals measured in minutes rather than hours, and peak flow before and after treatment where the patient can perform it. A patient too breathless to perform a peak flow has told you something, and the absence of a recorded value should be documented as inability rather than left blank.

Potassium requires monitoring in patients receiving repeated bronchodilators, which lower it, and this is a task that falls to nursing staff to prompt.

7.5 What Should Have Happened Sooner

The following is a composite case; identifying details have been changed.

Background

Kestrel had been diagnosed with asthma at the age of nine. In the 12 months before this admission she had attended an emergency department twice with asthma symptoms and had been discharged on both occasions without follow up being arranged. Her prescription record showed 11 reliever inhalers collected in that period and two preventer inhalers.

Presentation

Her presentation is described in section 7.1. What is not described there is that she delayed seeking help for approximately 14 hours, treating herself with escalating reliever doses through the night.

Analysis

Three risk factors were present and documented before she arrived. Emergency attendance without follow up, high reliever collection with low preventer collection, and delay in seeking help are each independently associated with fatal and near fatal asthma, and all three featured in the National Review of Asthma Deaths (Royal College of Physicians, 2014). None had generated any action. The enquiry recorded that 45 percent of people who died from asthma did not call for or receive medical assistance during their final attack, which is the statistical shape of Kestrel's 14 hours.

Intervention

Acute management is described in section 7.1. Before discharge she received a personal asthma action plan, a switch to a maintenance and reliever regimen, verified inhaler technique, and a respiratory clinic appointment at four weeks. Her general practice was contacted directly rather than by discharge letter alone.

Outcome

She attended the four week appointment. She did not attend the follow up arranged at six months. Her prescription record at one year showed three reliever inhalers and 10 combination inhalers, which is a substantial improvement and not a resolution.

Teaching Points

The risk factors that predicted this admission were visible in her records before she arrived and required no clinical judgment to identify, only somebody to look.

Guidance recommends that follow up be arranged after every emergency attendance for an asthma attack. Two previous opportunities to interrupt this trajectory were missed at exactly that point.

Improvement in a high risk patient is usually partial. Attendance at the first appointment and non attendance at the second is a common pattern and is not treatment failure.

7.6 The Attack That Looked Like Anxiety

The following account is a composite, with details changed for anonymity.

Zephyr, 19, presented to an emergency department at two in the morning, breathless, tearful, and hyperventilating, with a documented history of anxiety and a history of asthma described in the notes as mild childhood asthma. The triage entry recorded probable panic attack.

The nurse who assessed him took a peak flow, which he managed with difficulty, and it was 41 percent of his predicted value. That single measurement reclassified the presentation as acute severe asthma before any other assessment had been completed.

The complicating feature is that both things were true. He was having a panic attack, and he was having an asthma attack, and the panic was an entirely reasonable response to the asthma. Treating either in isolation would have been inadequate.

What the nurse did next is the part worth copying. She said that his chest was tight and that she was going to treat that first, that the frightened feeling was expected and would ease as his breathing did, and that she would stay. She did not attempt to talk him out of the anxiety and she did not treat the anxiety as the diagnosis.

He responded to standard treatment and was discharged the following afternoon. The notes from the admission recorded acute severe asthma. They did not record that the initial impression had been panic, and the triage entry was never reviewed. Nobody involved learned anything from an error that had been corrected within nine minutes by a peak flow reading, which is how most near misses in this field disappear.

Teaching points:

A psychiatric history in a breathless young patient increases rather than decreases the need for objective measurement.

Anxiety and asthma frequently coexist during an attack, and acknowledging the fear while treating the airway works better than addressing either alone.

7.7 The Window Before Discharge

The period between recovery and discharge is where the next attack is either prevented or arranged, and on a busy ward it is the period most likely to be compressed into a bag of medicines and a letter.

Four things need to happen and none of them requires a prescriber. Inhaler technique must be verified by demonstration, using the device the patient is actually going home with, as described in Chapter 5. A personal asthma action plan must be written with the patient's own doses on it and given to the patient rather than filed. The reason for the attack must be discussed, because a patient who cannot name what triggered this one has no way to avoid the next. And follow up must be arranged and confirmed rather than requested.

That last point carries specific weight in asthma. The National Review of Asthma Deaths recommended follow up after every emergency department or out of hours attendance for an attack, and Kestrel's history contains two attendances where that did not happen. A discharge letter asking a general practice to arrange review is a request. A booked appointment is an arrangement, and the difference between them is measurable in re attendance rates.

There is also a specific opportunity in the hours after a severe attack that does not exist at any other time. Patients who have been frightened are receptive in a way they are not at an annual review, and a conversation about preventer treatment held on the day after an attack lands differently from the same conversation held when the patient feels well. That is not a reason to be alarming. It is a reason not to defer the conversation to a clinic the patient may not attend.

Returning to the Start

At twenty five past three the registrar said that she sounded better. He was not careless and he was not inexperienced. He had arrived at that bed space with no knowledge of what the patient had sounded like at ten past, and the finding that mattered was not a sound but a change in a sound over 15 minutes.

That is the specific advantage the bedside nurse holds in acute asthma and it is not replicable by anyone arriving later. Continuity of observation converts a static finding into a trajectory, and in this condition the trajectory is the diagnosis. A quiet chest heard by someone who never heard the wheeze is an ambiguous finding. A quiet chest heard by someone who heard the wheeze 15 minutes earlier is an emergency.

What the nurse said, and what made the difference, was not a diagnosis. She said that the wheeze had gone but the patient had not improved, and that she thought the chest had gone quiet. Both halves of that sentence were required. The first reported a change, and the second named what she thought it meant, which gave the registrar something to disagree with specifically rather than a general expression of concern to reassure away.

Kestrel's admission had been predictable for a year, from a prescription record that nobody read and two emergency attendances that generated no follow up. The four minutes on the ward were where it was survived. The preventable part had already happened, months earlier, in a system that recorded 11 reliever inhalers and did nothing with the number.

Chapter 7 Review Questions

1. A patient with an acute asthma attack has a heart rate of 114 and is otherwise talking comfortably with a peak flow of 55 percent of predicted. How should this be graded?

A) Moderate, because the peak flow is above 50 percent and the patient is comfortable

B) Acute severe, because any single qualifying feature places the patient in that category

C) Life threatening, because tachycardia indicates cardiovascular compromise

D) The grade cannot be assigned without a blood gas

Answer: B. A heart rate of 110 or above is a defining feature of acute severe asthma. Features are not averaged, and a single qualifying feature determines the grade.

2. A patient with acute asthma has a blood gas showing a carbon dioxide level in the normal range. What does this indicate?

A) Adequate ventilation and a reassuring finding

B) Compensated respiratory acidosis

C) A near fatal attack, because carbon dioxide should be low in acute asthma

D) Sampling error requiring repeat

Answer: C. Patients with acute asthma hyperventilate, so carbon dioxide should be reduced. A normal or raised value indicates failing ventilation and places the attack in the near fatal category.

3. Which of the following was identified in the National Review of Asthma Deaths as a factor in a substantial proportion of fatal attacks?

A) Patients not calling for or receiving medical assistance during the final attack

B) Excessive use of spacer devices

C) Overuse of inhaled corticosteroids

D) Early referral to specialist services

Answer: A. The enquiry found that 45 percent of those who died did not call for or receive medical help during their final attack, which underlines the importance of action plans and of follow up after emergency attendance.

PART III: VENTILATORY SUPPORT ON THE WARD

Chapter 8: Starting Noninvasive Ventilation

Chapter Complexity Level: Advanced

Prerequisites: Chapters 2 and 3. Local noninvasive ventilation policy and competency framework.

Time Investment: Ninety minutes to read. One supervised set up to complete.

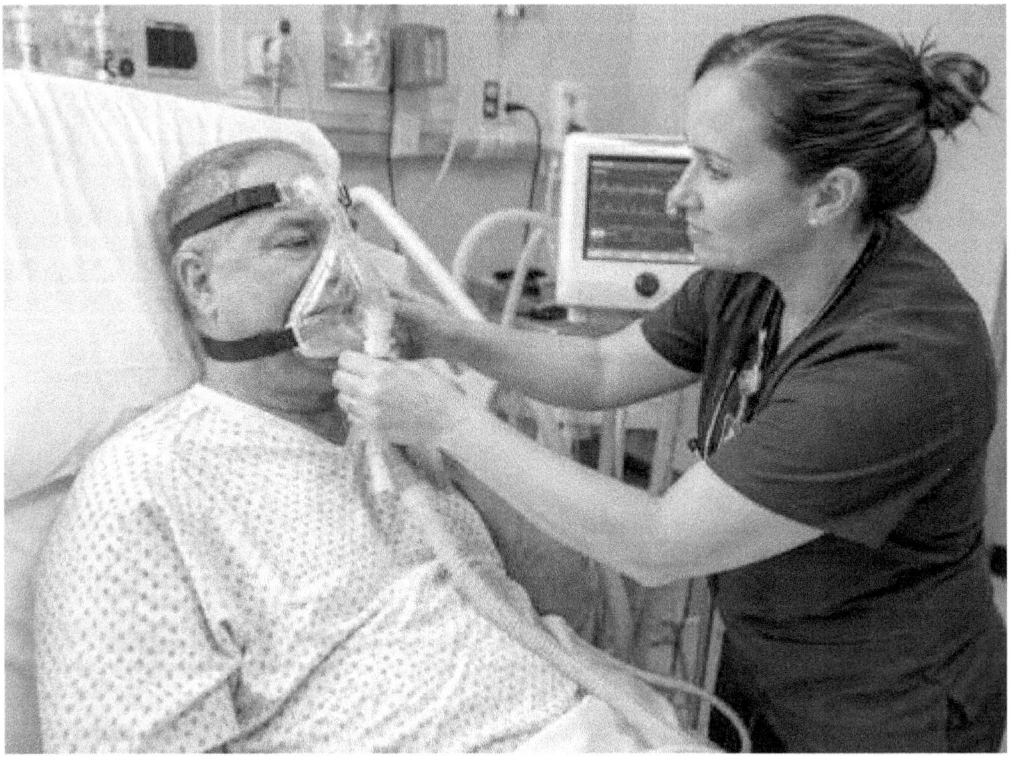

You have the gas in your hand. The pH is 7.27, the carbon dioxide is 9.2, the bicarbonate is 32, and you know from Chapter 3 exactly what that combination means. The machine is in the equipment room. You have watched it used perhaps four times, always by somebody else, and on two of those occasions the patient pulled the mask off within ten minutes. The registrar is in theatre. The patient is looking at you. What happens in the next hour will influence whether this admission ends in a discharge or an intensive care referral, and most of what determines it is nursing work.

8.1 What the Machine Is Doing

Noninvasive ventilation delivers pressure support through a mask rather than through a tube, and the two pressures it delivers do different jobs.

Inspiratory positive airway pressure, abbreviated to IPAP, is the pressure delivered during inhalation. It augments the patient's own breath, increases tidal volume, and therefore clears carbon dioxide. If carbon dioxide is the problem, IPAP is the answer.

Expiratory positive airway pressure, abbreviated to EPAP, is the pressure maintained during exhalation. It splints the airways open, recruits collapsed alveoli, and improves oxygenation. It also flushes exhaled gas from the mask and circuit.

The difference between the two pressures determines the ventilatory support. A machine set at 20 over 5 provides considerably more ventilation than one set at 12 over 8, even though the second has a higher expiratory pressure. Patients and relatives frequently assume the larger number is the important one. The gap between the numbers is what moves carbon dioxide.

Continuous positive airway pressure, or CPAP, delivers one pressure throughout the cycle. It improves oxygenation and reduces work of breathing but provides no ventilatory support, which means it does not clear carbon dioxide in the way bilevel ventilation does. Using CPAP in a hypercapnic patient is a recognised error and it is the reason the distinction matters at handover.

8.2 Deciding Whether to Start

The following worked example uses a composite case.

Dune, aged 77, has severe COPD and is admitted with an infective exacerbation. On arrival his gas shows a pH of 7.31, a carbon dioxide of 8.1, and a bicarbonate of 33. He is breathless, alert, and orientated.

Step one, does he meet the criteria. Persistent respiratory acidosis with hypercapnia despite medical therapy is the established indication for acute noninvasive ventilation in exacerbations of COPD (Davidson et al., 2016). His numbers sit in that territory.

Step two, what should happen first. The instinct to start immediately is wrong here, and the reason is well documented. Standard medical therapy comes first, including controlled oxygen targeted to 88 to 92 percent, nebulised bronchodilators, corticosteroids and antibiotics. A proportion of patients presenting with acidosis correct within the first hour on these measures alone.

Starting ventilation on a patient who would have corrected without it commits them to an uncomfortable intervention and occupies a resource.

Step three, the interval. Medical therapy is optimised and the gas is repeated after one hour. This is the step most often lost. The national confidential enquiry into acute noninvasive ventilation found a delay in initiating treatment in 27 percent of patients, with organisational factors and failure to recognise the indication both contributing (National Confidential Enquiry into Patient Outcome and Death, 2017). The repeat gas at one hour is the mechanism that prevents a planned interval from becoming an indefinite one.

Step four, the decision. Dune's repeat gas shows a pH of 7.28 and a carbon dioxide of 8.6. He has not corrected and he has deteriorated slightly. Ventilation is indicated.

The complicating moment. Before the machine is connected, one further question needs an answer, and it is the question most often deferred. If ventilation fails, what happens next. Is this patient a candidate for intubation, or is noninvasive ventilation the ceiling of treatment. That decision belongs to a senior clinician and it must be made and documented before the mask goes on rather than at four in the morning when it fails. Chapter 10 covers this in full. The nursing task at this point is to ask the question aloud and ensure the answer is recorded.

What this shows. Two of the four steps were about timing rather than technique, and the fourth was about a conversation. The equipment was the smallest part of the decision.

8.3 Preparing the Patient

Tolerance is established before the mask touches the face, and the preparation takes about 90 seconds.

Explain what the machine does in terms of the patient's own experience rather than in terms of pressures. It will push air in and it will feel strange at first. It will make breathing easier, not harder, once they stop fighting it. They can have it removed if they need to, and somebody will be with them.

That last point does more for tolerance than any other. A patient who believes the mask is being fixed to them will resist it. A patient who believes it can come off will usually leave it on.

Sit the patient upright. Position affects both the mechanics of ventilation and the patient's sense of control, and a patient lying flat with a mask on their face is being ventilated in the least comfortable and least effective posture available.

Hold the mask against the face by hand for the first minute or two before applying the straps at all. This single practice, letting the patient feel the pressure while retaining the ability to move away from it, prevents a substantial proportion of early intolerance.

> **Teaching Point:** *The commonest reason a patient does not tolerate noninvasive ventilation is not the pressure. It is the sensation of having something strapped to the face while frightened and unable to breathe. Time spent on the first two minutes buys more than any adjustment made in the following hour.*

8.4 Fitting the Mask

Mask selection and fit determine leak, comfort, and pressure damage, and all three determine whether the treatment works.

Size using the manufacturer's gauge rather than by eye. The commonest fitting error is selecting a mask that is too large, on the reasoning that a bigger mask will leak less. It leaks more, because it does not sit on the facial contours it was designed for.

Strap tension is the second error and it runs in the same direction. Overtightening does not eliminate leak and it does cause pressure damage. The conventional check is that two fingers should pass comfortably under the straps. A mask that leaks at appropriate tension is the wrong mask or the wrong size, and tightening it further converts one problem into two.

Protect the bridge of the nose from the beginning rather than when redness appears. A hydrocolloid or foam dressing applied before the mask goes on for the first time is standard practice in units that have low rates of device related pressure damage, and it is a nursing decision that requires nobody's permission.

Inspect the skin at every set of observations. Pressure damage from a ventilation mask develops in hours rather than days, and the patient cannot tell you it is happening because they cannot feel the difference between pressure and pressure.

8.5 The First Hour

The first hour determines the outcome and the observations during it are almost entirely nursing observations.

Starting pressures follow local protocol. Guidance describes commencing at a lower inspiratory pressure and titrating upward according to clinical response, respiratory rate, and blood gases, rather than starting at the target pressure (Davidson et al., 2016). Patients tolerate a gradual increase considerably better than an abrupt one, and a machine set correctly on a patient who will not wear it is delivering nothing.

Record the settings, the mask type and size, the patient's respiratory rate, their level of consciousness, their comfort, and the presence and site of any leak. Settings that are not recorded cannot be titrated, and a machine display read once at set up tells the next shift nothing about what has changed.

The repeat gas is the critical measurement. It should be taken at approximately one hour after starting, and the pH is the value that matters. A rising pH indicates the treatment is working. A static or falling pH after an hour of adequately delivered ventilation is a failure signal and requires senior review at that point rather than at the next routine gas.

Two clinical observations carry as much weight as the gas. A falling respiratory rate alongside improving comfort and maintained alertness is improvement. A falling respiratory rate alongside increasing drowsiness is deterioration, and it is the same distinction that Chapters 1 and 7 have now established in three separate contexts because it is the one most often misread.

8.6 When Not to Start

Contraindications matter because the harm from ventilating the wrong patient is immediate rather than gradual.

Absolute contraindications are few and they are mostly about the airway. A patient who cannot protect their own airway, who has severe facial trauma or recent upper airway surgery, who has a fixed upper airway obstruction, or who has vomited and is at risk of aspirating should not receive mask ventilation. An untreated pneumothorax is a further absolute contraindication until it has been drained, because positive pressure applied to an undrained pneumothorax can enlarge it rapidly.

Relative contraindications require a judgment rather than a rule. Confusion and agitation reduce tolerance but are also frequently caused by the hypercapnia that ventilation treats, which makes them a reason for closer supervision rather than automatic exclusion. Copious secretions are a genuine problem, because a mask impedes clearance, and a patient who is drowning in sputum needs the clearance addressed alongside the ventilation. Haemodynamic instability tolerates positive pressure poorly.

The category that causes most difficulty on a general ward is the patient with hypoxaemic rather than hypercapnic respiratory failure. Noninvasive ventilation has a much weaker evidence base in that group, and where it is used it should be in an environment where intubation can happen immediately, because hypoxaemia can develop within seconds if the mask is displaced. Applying mask ventilation to a hypoxaemic patient on a general ward, in the hope of avoiding an intensive care referral, is a recognised pattern and it delays a decision rather than avoiding it.

Aspiration risk deserves one specific note. Patients should not eat while receiving mask ventilation, and where treatment is prolonged, nutrition needs a plan rather than an assumption that breaks in therapy will provide it.

8.7 The Patient Who Would Not Keep It On

The following account is a composite, with details changed for anonymity.

Solstice, aged 81, was started on noninvasive ventilation at eleven at night. Within 20 minutes she had pulled the mask off three times. She was described in the notes as non compliant and the night team discussed whether to abandon the attempt.

The nurse who took over at midnight did three things before touching the settings. She checked the mask size against the gauge and found it was one size too large, which had been selected because the correct size had not been available on the ward at the time. She noted that Solstice had been laid flat when the mask was applied. And she asked Solstice what was actually wrong, and received an answer nobody had elicited, which was that the air was blowing into her eyes.

Leak directed at the eyes is a recognised consequence of poor mask fit, it is intensely uncomfortable, and it is not a form of non compliance. The correct mask was located from another ward, the patient was sat upright, and she tolerated the following six hours without difficulty.

It would be tidy to end there. In fact Solstice's pH improved only marginally over the next 12 hours and she was transferred to a higher level of care the following afternoon. The mask problem was real and correcting it was necessary, and it did not turn out to be the only thing that was wrong. The label of non compliance, however, would have concealed both.

Teaching points:

The word non compliant, applied to a patient on ventilation, is almost always a description of an unsolved equipment or communication problem.

Asking the patient what is wrong precedes adjusting the machine, and it is skipped most often with the patients least able to volunteer the answer.

Putting It to Work

The practical position is narrower than the physiology. Confirm that medical therapy has been optimised and that a gas has been repeated after an hour, because starting too early and starting too late are both common and the second is commoner. Establish before the mask goes on what happens if this fails, and make sure somebody has written it down.

Then spend your effort on the first two minutes rather than the settings. Hold the mask by hand. Sit the patient up. Size from the gauge, not by eye. Dress the nasal bridge before there is anything to dress. These are not comfort measures attached to a clinical intervention. In a treatment whose commonest mode of failure is that the patient will not wear it, they are the clinical intervention.

At one hour, look at the pH and look at the patient, and be clear which of the two possible falling respiratory rates you are seeing. If the pH has not moved, escalate then. The enquiry finding that care was suboptimal in more than 80 percent of reviewed cases did not describe a workforce that lacked machines. It described delays, unrecognised indications, inconsistent titration, and patients who never reached target pressures at all, which are failures of process occurring at the bedside over hours.

British Thoracic Society quality standards specify that all staff who prescribe, initiate or alter acute noninvasive ventilation should have evidence of training and maintenance of competence (Davies et al., 2018). Work within your local policy and your assessed competence throughout. This chapter explains what is happening and why so that you can recognise what you are looking at. It does not authorise you to set or change pressures outside the framework your employer has established.

Chapter 8 Review Questions

1. **A patient with an exacerbation of COPD has a pH of 7.30 and a carbon dioxide of 8.0 on arrival. What is the most appropriate initial management?**

A) Immediate commencement of noninvasive ventilation

B) Optimise medical therapy including controlled oxygen, then repeat the gas after approximately one hour

C) Increase inspired oxygen to correct the hypoxaemia first

D) Repeat the gas at the next routine round in four hours

Answer: B. A proportion of patients correct with medical therapy alone within the first hour. Option D is the commoner error in practice and converts a planned interval into a delay.

2. **Which pressure setting primarily determines carbon dioxide clearance?**

A) The expiratory pressure alone

B) The difference between inspiratory and expiratory pressures

C) The inspired oxygen concentration

D) The back up rate alone

Answer: B. Ventilation, and therefore carbon dioxide clearance, is driven by the pressure support delivered, which is the gap between the two pressures rather than either value alone.

3. **A patient repeatedly removes the ventilation mask within minutes of application. What should be assessed before the settings are altered?**

A) Whether sedation is required

B) Mask size and fit, patient position, and what specifically the patient reports as the problem

C) Whether the patient has capacity to refuse treatment

D) Whether the inspiratory pressure should be increased to improve efficacy

Answer: B. Early intolerance is most often caused by an oversized mask, poor positioning, or leak directed at the eyes. Increasing pressure in an intolerant patient reliably worsens the problem.

Chapter 9: Troubleshooting Ventilation Failure

Chapter Complexity Level: Advanced

Prerequisites: Chapter 8. Local noninvasive ventilation policy.

Time Investment: Ninety minutes to read. Three simulated deteriorations to work through.

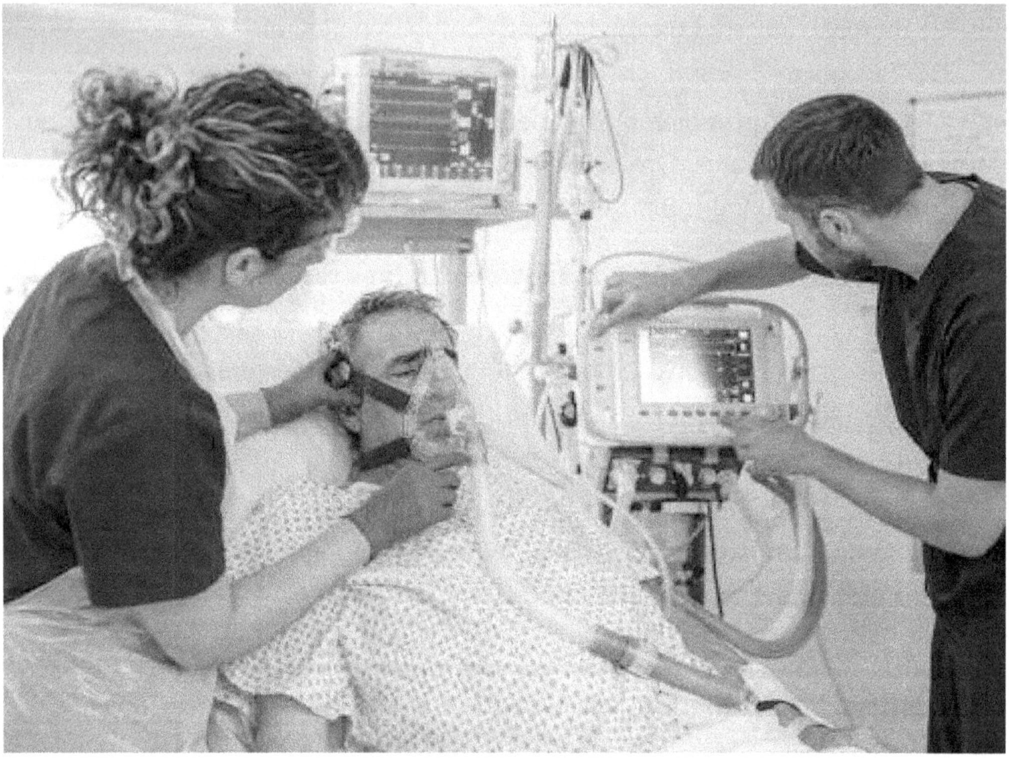

Umber and Ellis were started on noninvasive ventilation within an hour of each other on the same ward, both with exacerbations of COPD, both with a pH just below 7.30, both on the same model of machine at similar settings. Six hours later Umber was comfortable, his pH was 7.36, and the plan was to wean him overnight. Ellis had been transferred to intensive care. The difference was not the diagnosis, the machine, or the pressures. It was what happened during two separate episodes in the second hour, when each patient became distressed and the alarm sounded, and what the nurse present decided the alarm meant.

9.1 The Problem With the Word Failure

Ventilation that is not working attracts a single label, and the label conceals four entirely different problems with four different remedies.

The mask may be wrong, in size, type, or position. The circuit may be leaking, disconnected, or obstructed. The settings may be inadequate for the patient's requirement, or inappropriate for their breathing pattern. Or the patient may be deteriorating despite adequately delivered ventilation, which is the only one of the four that means the treatment has failed.

Collapsing all four into failure produces two opposite errors. Patients get escalated to intensive care for a problem that a different mask would have solved. And patients who are genuinely deteriorating get another 90 minutes of adjustment while somebody works through the equipment, because the equipment is the thing that can be fiddled with.

The national confidential enquiry found ventilator settings titrated inconsistently and 45 percent of patients not reaching target pressures at all (National Confidential Enquiry into Patient Outcome and Death, 2017). A figure of that size is not explained by machines breaking. It describes a delivery problem occurring at the bedside, hour after hour, on wards where the treatment was correctly indicated and correctly prescribed.

9.2 Why Protocols Have Not Solved It

Most units have a noninvasive ventilation protocol. Most protocols specify indications, starting pressures, and escalation criteria, and stop there.

What protocols rarely specify is what to do in the third hour when the patient is distressed, the machine is alarming, and the numbers on the screen do not match the numbers that were recorded at set up. That is the moment where the enquiry's findings are generated, and it is a diagnostic moment rather than a protocol moment.

The second gap is training design, and it repeats the pattern described in Chapter 5. Noninvasive ventilation training is typically delivered once, on a machine that may not be the machine on the ward, to staff who then encounter the situation infrequently. British Thoracic Society quality standards require evidence of training and maintained competence for all staff who initiate or alter acute ventilation (Davies et al., 2018), which is a standard about currency rather than attendance, and currency is what a single induction session does not provide.

9.3 Four Questions in Order

When ventilation appears not to be working, ask these four questions in this order. The order is deliberate, moving from the most common and most correctable to the least.

Is it the interface? Look at the mask before anything else. Size, position, strap tension, and the direction of any audible leak. A leak into the eyes, described in section 8.7, produces distress that looks like intolerance of ventilation and is intolerance of something else entirely.

Is it the circuit? Follow the tubing from the machine to the patient with your hands. Disconnection, kinking under bedding, water accumulation in the tubing, an occluded or absent expiratory port. Exhalation ports are not optional and covering one causes rebreathing.

Is it the settings? Compare the machine display against the settings recorded at set up. Look at the delivered tidal volume and the leak figure if the machine displays them. A patient whose requirement has increased may be receiving adequate pressure for the patient they were three hours ago.

Is it the patient? Only when the first three have been excluded does distress become a clinical rather than a technical finding. At that point it means deterioration and it needs escalation, not adjustment.

> **Teaching Point:** *The order protects against the commonest error, which is going straight to question four and escalating a mask problem, and against its mirror image, which is remaining stuck on questions one to three while a patient deteriorates. Work through them quickly, but work through them.*

9.4 Leak and Asynchrony

The following worked example uses a composite case.

Rumi, aged 69, has been on ventilation for two hours. She is increasingly distressed. The machine is alarming intermittently and the nurse notes that Rumi appears to be fighting the breaths rather than receiving them.

Step one, the interface. The mask is the correct size and appropriately positioned. There is an audible leak at the left cheek. The straps are already tight.

Step two, the reasoning. Tightening further is the obvious response and it is the wrong one. Leak at one side with a correctly sized mask usually indicates asymmetric positioning or a distorted cushion rather than insufficient tension, and the correct action is to release the straps, reseat the mask, and retension evenly. This is done, and the leak reduces substantially.

Step three, what remains. Rumi is still fighting the breaths. Watching her chest against the machine, the nurse observes that Rumi begins to exhale while the machine is still delivering inspiratory pressure, and that some of her inspiratory efforts do not trigger a breath at all.

Step four, naming it. This is **asynchrony**, which means the machine and the patient are working to different rhythms. Ineffective triggering, where the patient's effort fails to initiate a breath, and cycling that does not match the patient's own inspiratory time are the two commonest forms and both are visible at the bedside without waveform expertise. Watch the patient's chest and abdomen and listen to the machine. If the two are not in step, they are not in step.

The complicating moment. The nurse's competency framework does not permit her to adjust the trigger sensitivity or the inspiratory time. What it does permit, and what she does, is to document precisely what she has observed, correct the leak that was contributing to the ineffective triggering, and request review with a specific description rather than a general report of distress. Leak is a common cause of asynchrony because leaked volume is interpreted by the machine as continuing inspiratory flow, so correcting the interface frequently corrects the synchrony without any settings change at all.

What this shows. Two of the four questions were answered before anyone considered the patient to be failing. Neither required a prescriber. The description handed over was specific enough for a decision to be made by somebody who had not been in the room.

9.5 Pressure Damage and Other Costs

Ventilation causes harm even when it works, and most of that harm is preventable by nursing action.

Device related pressure damage to the nasal bridge is the commonest and it develops in hours. Prevention, as described in section 8.4, is prophylactic dressing from the outset and skin inspection at every observation set. When damage appears despite this, the answer is a change of interface rather than a change of dressing. Rotating between a full face mask and a nasal mask, or moving to a total face mask or helmet where available, transfers the pressure to different tissue.

Gastric distension results from air entering the oesophagus at higher pressures. It causes discomfort, splints the diaphragm, and increases aspiration risk. It is worth reporting rather than tolerating.

Dryness of the mouth, nose, and eyes is close to universal at higher flows and is a frequent driver of the intolerance discussed in Chapter 8. Humidification, regular mouth care, and attention to leak direction address it. Patients rarely complain about it because they are preoccupied with breathing, and it is therefore something to ask about rather than wait for.

Sleep deprivation deserves more attention than it receives. A patient on ventilation in a bay, with alarms and hourly observations, may go 48 hours without meaningful sleep, and exhaustion is itself a cause of ventilatory failure. Clustering interventions and protecting periods of rest is a clinical decision in this population rather than a courtesy.

Communication loss is the cost patients themselves rate most highly and clinicians record least. A person wearing a full face mask cannot speak, cannot easily be understood when they try, and is frequently frightened. A pen and paper within reach, an agreed hand signal for take this off, and a habit of asking closed questions that can be answered with a nod are small provisions that change the experience substantially. Patients who have a means of being understood tolerate ventilation for longer, and the mechanism is not mysterious.

9.6 Two Alarms, Two Decisions

The following are composite cases.

Case A

Umber became distressed at 90 minutes and the low pressure alarm sounded. The nurse worked through the interface and found the mask had ridden upward, producing leak at the bridge and pressure on the eyes. She reseated it, resettled him upright, and stayed for four minutes while he settled. She documented the event and the correction. His pH at the four hour gas was 7.34 and continued to improve.

Case B

Ellis became distressed at 100 minutes. The nurse increased the inspiratory pressure, on the reasoning that a distressed patient needs more support. Distress increased. She then attributed the deterioration to intolerance and requested sedation, which was declined. By the time a senior review occurred at three hours, Ellis was drowsy with a rising carbon dioxide and was transferred.

Both nurses were competent and both responded promptly. The difference was the order of the questions. Umber's nurse asked what was wrong before deciding what to do about it. Ellis's nurse began with the response rather than the assessment, and the response she chose, increasing pressure in a distressed patient, reliably worsens tolerance. What could not be established afterwards, and this matters, is whether Ellis would have avoided transfer had the sequence been followed. He was sicker than Umber at the outset. The failure of process is clear. The counterfactual is not.

9.7 Weaning and Handover

Ventilation that is working eventually has to stop, and the weaning period generates its own set of avoidable readmissions to a higher level of care.

Weaning is usually achieved by progressively increasing the length of breaks rather than by reducing pressures, with overnight ventilation retained longest because carbon dioxide typically rises during sleep. A patient who has tolerated four hours off during the day has not demonstrated that they will tolerate a night off, and that distinction gets lost when a daytime team documents good tolerance and a night team reads it as readiness.

Three observations matter during breaks. Respiratory rate, conscious level, and how the patient looks toward the end of the break rather than at the start. A patient who is comfortable at 20 minutes and labouring at 90 has told you the duration is too long, and that information is only available to somebody who looks twice.

Handover deserves specific attention because ventilation is one of the few ward treatments where the settings can drift without anybody deciding to change them. A handover that states the patient is on noninvasive ventilation has communicated almost nothing. A useful handover states the current settings, the settings at commencement, the mask type and size, the time and result of the last gas, the current break schedule, the tolerance history, and crucially the documented ceiling of care.

That last item is the one most often absent, and its absence is what turns a deterioration at four in the morning into an argument rather than a plan. Chapter 10 takes up why it goes missing and what the conversation that fills the gap actually sounds like.

Where This Leaves Us

Three things are settled. Most apparent ventilation failure in the first hours is interface or circuit failure, not treatment failure, and it is correctable at the bedside by staff who do not need prescribing authority to correct it. Increasing pressure in a distressed patient is the wrong reflex and it makes tolerance worse. And a static or falling pH after an hour of adequately delivered ventilation is a genuine failure signal requiring senior review at that point.

What is not settled is more uncomfortable. The confidential enquiry evidence tells us that inconsistent titration and failure to reach target pressures were widespread. It does not tell us how many of those patients would have done better had delivery been optimal, because that comparison has not been made and probably cannot be made outside a trial. It is reasonable to believe that better delivery improves outcomes. It is not demonstrated that it accounts for the mortality signal that prompted the enquiry in the first place.

There is a second open question, which is whether the bedside distinctions in this chapter are reliably teachable. Recognising asynchrony by watching a chest is a skill that experienced respiratory nurses clearly possess and that has never been formally validated as a nursing observation. This chapter presents it because it is useful and because the alternative on a general ward at three in the morning is nothing at all. A reader should hold it with the confidence that clinical experience warrants and not more.

What is not in doubt is the order of the four questions, and that is the part to take onto a shift.

Chapter 9 Review Questions

1. **A patient on noninvasive ventilation becomes distressed at 90 minutes with an audible leak at one side of the mask, despite tight straps. What is the most appropriate action?**

A) Tighten the straps further to eliminate the leak

B) Increase the inspiratory pressure to compensate for the leak

C) Release the straps, reseat the mask, and retension evenly

D) Discontinue ventilation and request urgent review

Answer: C. Unilateral leak with a correctly sized mask usually reflects asymmetric positioning rather than inadequate tension. Further tightening causes pressure damage without correcting the leak.

2. **Which finding after one hour of adequately delivered ventilation most clearly indicates treatment failure requiring senior review?**

A) A persistent audible leak

B) A static or falling pH

C) A respiratory rate that has fallen from 30 to 24

D) Patient reports of dry mouth

Answer: B. The pH is the primary marker of response. A falling respiratory rate must be interpreted alongside conscious level, as a fall accompanied by increasing drowsiness indicates deterioration.

3. **Why can a significant mask leak cause ineffective triggering?**

A) It reduces the oxygen concentration delivered

B) Leaked volume may be interpreted by the machine as continuing inspiratory flow

C) It increases the expiratory pressure automatically

D) It causes the machine to switch to a back up rate

Answer: B. Because leak is misread as ongoing patient flow, correcting the interface frequently resolves asynchrony without any change to settings.

Chapter 10: When Ventilation Is the Ceiling

Chapter Complexity Level: Advanced

Prerequisites: Chapters 8 and 9.

Time Investment: One hour to read. One reflective exercise to complete.

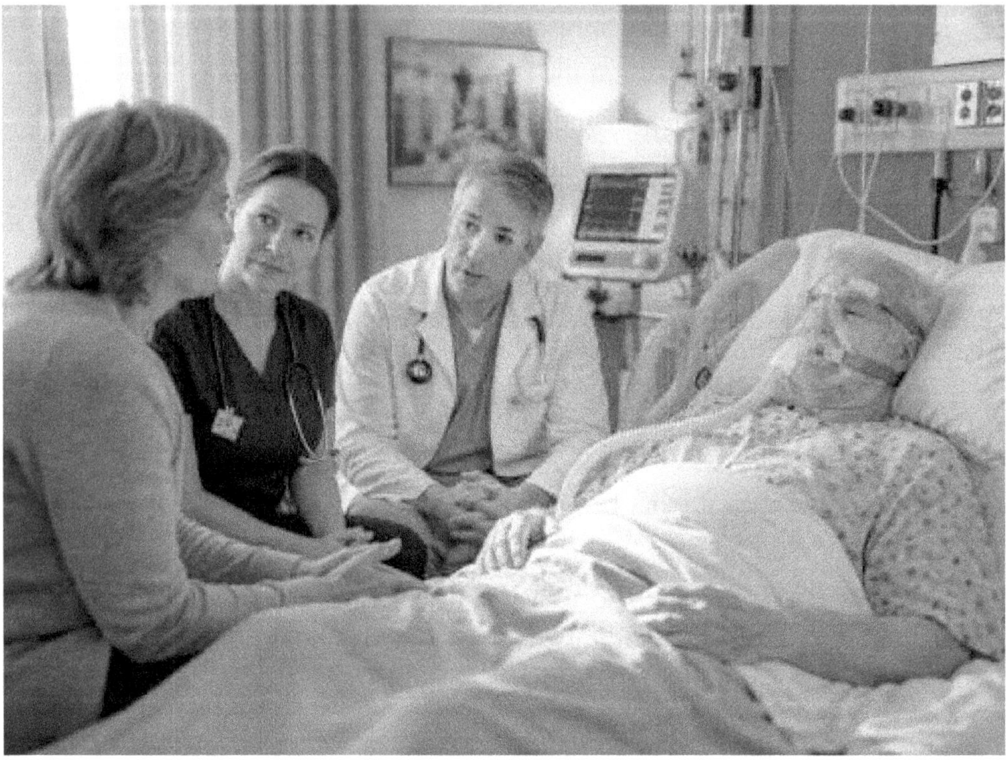

The field does not have a settled answer to the question of when noninvasive ventilation stops being a treatment and becomes a way of prolonging a death. Guidance supports its use as a ceiling of care in patients for whom intubation is not appropriate, and the evidence that it improves survival in that group is real. Guidance also acknowledges that some patients receive it for days while deteriorating, unable to speak to their families, in a treatment nobody has revisited. Both descriptions are accurate and they sometimes describe the same patient at different hours. This chapter examines a disagreement the literature has not resolved, and it does not resolve it either.

10.1 What Is Actually Disputed

The dispute is not about whether noninvasive ventilation should be offered to patients who are not candidates for intubation. That question has an answer, and the answer is that it should. Ventilation as a ceiling of treatment is an established position, it is supported by outcome data, and withholding it from a patient because they are not for intubation is a straightforward error.

What is disputed is narrower and harder. It concerns what should happen when a patient with ventilation as their ceiling is not improving. At that point the treatment has, by definition, no escalation above it. The available options are to continue, to continue with a defined review point, or to withdraw and move to symptom control.

Practice varies enormously. Some units review such patients formally at fixed intervals. Others continue until the patient dies wearing the mask. The difference is rarely documented as a decision and is more often the accumulated result of nobody deciding.

10.2 The Case for Persisting

The strongest version of the argument for continuing runs as follows.

Recovery from acute on chronic hypercapnic respiratory failure is not linear. Patients improve over days rather than hours, and a patient who has not improved at 12 hours may improve at 36. Withdrawing at the first plateau removes a treatment from patients who would have survived, and survival in this group is not marginal. Patients with exacerbations of COPD who receive ventilation as their ceiling of care have meaningful survival rates and many return to a quality of life they value (Davidson et al., 2016).

There is a second argument, which concerns who is making the judgment. Clinicians caring for people with severe chronic respiratory disease frequently rate those patients' quality of life lower than the patients rate it themselves, a discrepancy repeatedly described across chronic and life limiting illness. A clinician who concludes that continuing is not worthwhile may therefore be applying a standard the patient does not share. This is a well recognised clinical caution rather than a quantified effect, and it is offered here as a reason for humility rather than as a measurement.

The third argument is practical. Withdrawal decisions taken at night, by staff who do not know the patient, in the absence of family, are the worst possible circumstances for an irreversible choice. A bias toward continuing until a senior review can happen properly is defensible on those grounds alone.

10.3 The Case for Stopping

The strongest version of the argument for withdrawal is equally serious.

A patient who is dying and who is wearing a full face mask cannot speak to their family. Communication is the thing patients and relatives consistently identify as mattering most in the final days, and mask ventilation removes it almost entirely. A treatment that is not going to achieve recovery is, in that circumstance, exchanging a person's last conversations for hours of continued physiology.

Ventilation also has burdens that are easy to underestimate from outside. The mask is uncomfortable. Sleep is fragmented or absent. The patient cannot eat normally, cannot be easily held, and is frequently frightened. Those burdens are acceptable in exchange for recovery and become difficult to justify without it.

There is a further consideration about honesty. Continuing a treatment because nobody has revisited it is not the same as continuing it because it has been judged appropriate, and families are frequently told the first while believing the second. A relative who understands the mask as a cure will interpret its continuation as evidence of hope, and will experience its eventual removal as abandonment rather than as a change of goal.

10.4 What the Evidence Supports and Where It Stops

The evidence base supports several specific propositions and runs out before it reaches the question this chapter is about.

It supports the use of ventilation in patients not suitable for intubation, and it supports meaningful survival in that group. It supports the position that decisions about escalation should be made before the treatment starts rather than during a crisis, and this is where the confidential enquiry evidence is most directly relevant. Where a ceiling has not been documented in advance, the decision falls to whoever is present at the moment of deterioration, which is usually a junior doctor and a ward nurse at an unsociable hour with no family present.

What the evidence does not supply is a threshold. There is no validated point at which continued ventilation in a non improving patient becomes futile, no score, and no interval. Clinical judgment fills that space, and clinical judgment in this territory is influenced by the composition of the team on duty and by how the conversation was framed on admission.

> **Teaching Point:** *The decision that reliably prevents the worst version of this situation is made before ventilation starts, not during it. A documented ceiling of care and a documented review point convert a crisis judgment into a planned one, and the nurse setting up the machine is well placed to ask for both.*

10.5 What a Nurse Actually Does

Whatever position a practitioner holds, several actions follow that do not depend on resolving the debate.

Ask for the ceiling to be documented before the mask goes on, as described in section 8.2. Ask what the review point is and what would constitute improvement, so that a plan exists against which the next 24 hours can be assessed.

Establish what the family understands. This is the highest value nursing action in the whole chapter and it takes one question, which is what they have been told about what the machine is doing. The answers reveal the gap between what was said and what was heard, and the gap is frequently large.

Protect communication while it is still possible. A patient with a documented ceiling who is not improving may have a window of hours in which they can still speak. Arranging breaks in therapy specifically so that a person can talk to their family is a legitimate clinical decision, not a compromise of treatment, and it requires somebody to think of it early.

And describe the burdens accurately when the review happens. The team deciding whether to continue needs to know that the patient has not slept, has pulled the mask off nine times, and asked this morning whether he was going to die. That information exists only at the bedside.

10.6 Two Families, Two Understandings

The following are composite cases.

Case A

Nyx, aged 84, was started on ventilation with a documented ceiling. The nurse asked his daughter what she understood the machine to be doing. The daughter said it was helping him breathe while the antibiotics worked, and that he would come off it when he was better. That was broadly accurate and it omitted the ceiling entirely. The nurse arranged for the medical team to speak with the family that evening. When Nyx did not improve over the following two days, the conversation about withdrawal took place with a family who already understood the plan. He died with the mask off, in the presence of his daughter and his son.

Case B

Bellamy, aged 79, was started on ventilation on a Friday evening with no documented ceiling. Over the weekend he did not improve. Each shift continued the treatment, reasonably, in the absence of any plan to the contrary. The conversation with his family took place on Monday morning, initiated because a consultant reviewed him and asked why he was still on it. His wife had spent three days believing the machine was curing him. He died that afternoon. His wife said afterwards that nobody had told her he was dying, and she was right.

The clinical trajectories were similar. The difference was that one family had been given time to arrive at an understanding and the other had it delivered to them in a single conversation at the end. Neither team acted wrongly at any individual moment. Bellamy's weekend was made of defensible decisions by people who did not know a decision was being made.

10.7 The Conversation Nobody Scheduled

The following account is a composite, with details changed for anonymity.

Cypress had been a respiratory nurse for six years and described the part of the job she had found hardest as knowing what to say when a patient asked whether they were dying.

Her early strategy had been to redirect. She would say that the doctors were doing everything they could and that they should focus on getting through today. She described it later as a way of managing her own discomfort rather than the patient's, and as something patients saw through immediately.

What she moved to was slower and shorter. When a patient asked, she would ask what had made them think about it. The answers were usually specific. One man said he had noticed his family had stopped talking about next week. Another said he could feel it was different this time. Those answers gave her something to respond to that was true, and she found she could then say that she did not know how long, that she could see he was very unwell, and that she would find out what the medical team thought and come back.

The part she found she could not fix was the timing. The patients who asked her were frequently asking at two in the morning, when there was nobody to consult and no possibility of arranging a family conversation before the shift ended. She said that she had learned to write down exactly what the patient had asked and exactly what she had answered, and to hand it over verbally as well as in the notes, because otherwise the question disappeared with her at eight o'clock.

Teaching points:

Asking what prompted the question converts an unanswerable enquiry into a specific one that can be answered honestly.

A question asked at night is lost unless it is actively handed over, and it is frequently the most important thing that happened on the shift.

10.8 Withdrawing the Mask

When the decision has been made, the withdrawal itself is a nursing procedure and it goes better when it has been planned rather than improvised.

Symptom control comes first and comes before the mask comes off, not after. Anticipatory medication for breathlessness and distress should be prescribed and available at the bedside in advance, and the approaches described in Chapter 14 apply directly. A withdrawal that begins with the mask and then sends somebody to find a prescriber has been sequenced backwards.

Timing should accommodate the family rather than the drug round. If a daughter is two hours away, two hours is usually available. Ask who the patient would want present, and ask the family whether they wish to be in the room, making clear that either answer is reasonable and that they can change their mind.

Prepare people for what they will see. Breathing will change. It may become noisier or more irregular. The patient may appear more settled rather than less, which frequently surprises families who have been told the machine was helping. Saying this in advance prevents a distressing change from being interpreted as a mistake.

Remove the mask gently and attend to the face. Skin under a mask is frequently marked, sometimes broken, and always indented. Washing the face, offering mouth care, and repositioning pillows are not cosmetic acts at this point. They return a person to their family looking like themselves, and relatives remember it.

Afterwards, the team needs something too. Staff who have delivered intensive treatment for days and then withdrawn it carry that, and units where nobody ever debriefs are units where the same conversation happens privately in a corridor instead.

The Open Questions

The disagreement described in this chapter has not been resolved and this chapter has not resolved it. What can be stated is that the argument for persisting rests on real survival data and on well documented clinician bias about quality of life, and that the argument for stopping rests on burdens that are systematically underestimated and on a communication loss that is total while the mask is on. Anyone who finds one of those arguments obviously correct has probably not spent enough time with the other.

What is settled is that the decision belongs before the treatment rather than during it, that families need to understand the ceiling while there is still time for that understanding to develop, and that the burdens of treatment are visible mainly to nursing staff and therefore reportable mainly by them.

Which leaves a question worth sitting with, and it is not the one about futility. Bellamy's weekend consisted of a series of individually reasonable decisions by staff who did not know they were making one. Nobody chose to continue. The treatment simply carried on because it had started, and the absence of a review point meant that continuing required no decision while stopping would have required a considerable one.

So the question is this. In your own unit, what would have to change for the default to run the other way, so that continuing a treatment past a defined review point required somebody to decide it, and how much of that change is within the reach of the nurse who sets the machine up on a Friday evening?

Chapter 10 Review Questions

1. **A patient with severe COPD is not considered suitable for intubation. What is the appropriate position regarding noninvasive ventilation?**

A) It should be withheld, as there is no escalation available if it fails

B) It is an established treatment option in this group and should be considered

C) It should only be used with continuous critical care supervision

D) It should be offered only if the family requests it

Answer: B. Ventilation as a ceiling of treatment is well established and supported by outcome data. Withholding it because the patient is not for intubation is an error.

2. **When should a ceiling of care decision ideally be made and documented for a patient commencing noninvasive ventilation?**

A) At the point of deterioration, when the clinical picture is clearest

B) Before ventilation is commenced

C) At the first consultant ward round after commencement

D) Only if the patient asks about it

Answer: B. Deciding in advance converts a crisis judgment made by whoever is present into a planned one. Its absence is a recurring finding in reviews of ventilation care.

3. **Which nursing action most reliably reduces the risk of a family experiencing withdrawal of ventilation as abandonment?**

A) Ensuring the patient is comfortable throughout

B) Establishing early what the family understands the machine to be doing

C) Documenting the settings accurately at each shift

D) Delaying the conversation until the medical team is certain

Answer: B. The gap between what families are told and what they understand is frequently large, and identifying it early allows understanding to develop over days rather than being delivered in a single conversation at the end.

PART IV: SUPPURATIVE AND FIBROTIC LUNG DISEASE

Chapter 11: Bronchiectasis and Airway Clearance

Chapter Complexity Level: Intermediate

Prerequisites: Chapters 1 and 2.

Time Investment: One hour to read. One clearance session to teach.

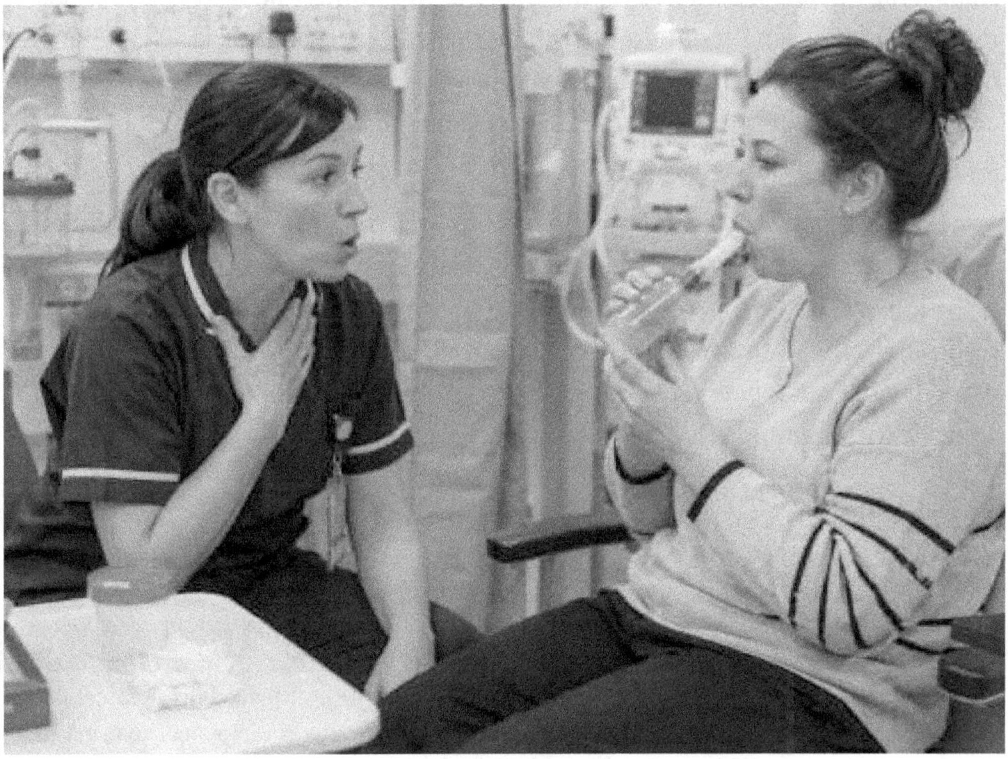

A respiratory physiotherapist once described bronchiectasis to a group of ward nurses as the only common respiratory condition where the most effective treatment is something the patient has to do rather than something anyone gives them. She meant it as an argument for spending time on technique. She was also, without intending to, explaining why bronchiectasis is managed less consistently than asthma or chronic obstructive disease on most general wards. A treatment that is administered has a drug round attached to it. A treatment the patient performs has nothing attached to it at all unless somebody builds the structure.

11.1 The Cycle That Sustains Itself

Bronchiectasis is permanent abnormal dilatation of the airways, and the clinical problem it produces is a cycle rather than a static defect.

Damaged airways clear secretions poorly. Retained secretions become colonised by bacteria. Bacterial presence provokes inflammation. Inflammation damages the airway wall further, which worsens clearance. Each turn of the cycle makes the next turn easier.

That model explains why clearance is treatment rather than comfort. Removing secretions interrupts the cycle at the point where the patient has most influence, and doing it daily rather than during exacerbations is what changes the trajectory. It also explains why a patient who feels well and stops clearing will deteriorate over months rather than days, which makes the connection between the behaviour and the consequence difficult for patients to perceive.

The British Thoracic Society guideline recommends that adults with bronchiectasis who have a chronic productive cough or difficulty with sputum retention should be offered personalised airway clearance techniques taught by a respiratory physiotherapist (Hill et al., 2019). The word personalised is doing real work in that sentence. Techniques are not interchangeable and patients do not comply with methods that do not suit them.

11.2 Techniques and Who They Suit

Technique	What it involves	Best suited to
Active cycle of breathing techniques	Cycles of breathing control, thoracic expansion exercises, and forced expiration	Most adults. Requires no equipment. The usual first choice
Autogenic drainage	Breathing at varying lung volumes to mobilise secretions from small to large airways	Patients who find forced expiration exhausting or who bronchospasm with huffing
Positive expiratory pressure devices	Exhaling against resistance, with or without oscillation	Patients who prefer a device to a technique, or who struggle to self direct
Postural drainage	Gravity assisted positioning	Adjunct where secretions are localised. Contraindicated or poorly tolerated in reflux, obesity, and cardiac disease

Two practical points determine whether any of these work.

The forced expiration, or huff, is the component patients most often perform incorrectly. It is a forced exhalation with an open glottis, not a cough. It should sound like breathing hard onto a mirror. Patients who convert it into a cough exhaust themselves, raise intrathoracic pressure, and clear less.

And the duration matters more than the elegance. A clearance session that lasts three minutes because the patient has somewhere to be is a session that has not reached the peripheral secretions. Ten to 20 minutes, once or twice daily, is the usual expectation, and a patient who does not know this will assume a brief session is adequate.

11.3 Getting the Order Right

The following worked example uses a composite case.

Yael, aged 58, has bronchiectasis and has been performing clearance daily for two years with little benefit. She is admitted with an exacerbation. Her prescription includes a bronchodilator, nebulised hypertonic saline, and a clearance regimen.

Step one, what she reports. She performs her clearance first thing in the morning. She uses the nebulised saline afterwards, because she was told it helps loosen secretions and she assumed that meant it prepared her for the following day.

Step two, why this fails. The sequence is inverted. Hyperosmolar agents such as nebulised hypertonic saline draw water into the airway and reduce sputum viscosity, and guidance describes using them before physiotherapy clearance to mobilise secretions in patients with high sputum volume or tenacious secretions (Hill et al., 2019). Used afterwards, the agent thins secretions that are then left in place until the following morning.

Step three, the corrected sequence. Bronchodilator first, which opens the airway and reduces the bronchospasm that hypertonic saline can provoke. Then the hyperosmolar agent. Then clearance, promptly while the secretions are mobilised. Then, where prescribed, inhaled antibiotic last, delivered into an airway that has just been cleared so the drug reaches the surface it is meant to treat.

The complicating moment. Yael reports that hypertonic saline makes her cough violently and that she has sometimes skipped it. This is a recognised effect rather than intolerance in the sense of a reason to stop, and a bronchodilator beforehand and a test dose with monitoring are the standard responses. The nurse's instinct to reassure her that it is harmless would be accurate and unhelpful. What she does instead is document the reaction, ensure the bronchodilator is given first, and ask the medical team to review whether the concentration is appropriate.

What this shows. Nothing was added to Yael's treatment. The same four items were reordered, and the reordering is the intervention. Sequence errors of this kind persist for years because each individual component is prescribed correctly and nobody asks the patient in what order she does them.

> **Teaching Point:** *Ask any patient with bronchiectasis to describe their morning in order, from waking. Sequence errors are invisible on a drug chart and obvious in 60 seconds of description.*

11.4 Sputum as Data

Sputum is the most informative and least systematically recorded observation in bronchiectasis nursing.

Three properties carry information. Volume, which patients can estimate in familiar terms such as a teaspoon or an egg cup. Colour, which ranges from clear through cream to yellow, green, and brown, with increasing purulence indicating increasing inflammation and bacterial load. And viscosity, which affects clearability directly.

The clinically useful measurement is change from that patient's own baseline, which means the baseline has to be known. A patient who habitually produces a cupful of green sputum every morning is not exacerbating because they produced a cupful of green sputum this morning. A patient who normally produces a teaspoon of cream coloured sputum and is now producing green sputum has changed, and change is the signal.

Sampling has its own requirements. Send a sample before antibiotics start rather than after, take it in the morning when the overnight accumulation is being cleared, and take it after a clearance session rather than before, because a sample of saliva reported as no growth is worse than no sample at all. Patients with bronchiectasis frequently have established colonisation, and knowing which organism is present shapes both the acute and the long term antibiotic decision.

11.5 Long Term Treatment and Its Monitoring

Patients with frequent exacerbations may be on long term macrolide antibiotics or inhaled antibiotics, and both carry monitoring obligations that fall largely to nursing and primary care.

Long term macrolides require that non tuberculous mycobacterial infection has been excluded before starting, because macrolide monotherapy in that context promotes resistance. They also require attention to hearing, liver function, and cardiac conduction. Patients rarely know why they are having these checks, and a patient who does not know why a test is being done is a patient who stops attending for it.

Inhaled antibiotics commonly provoke bronchospasm, particularly with the first dose, which is why an initial dose is usually given under observation with lung function measured before and after. A bronchodilator beforehand is standard.

Adherence is the recurring problem and it deserves an honest framing. A patient with bronchiectasis may be asked to perform twice daily clearance, use a nebulised agent, take an inhaled antibiotic, and attend for monitoring bloods, indefinitely, while feeling reasonably well. Treating non adherence as a knowledge deficit misdiagnoses it. The realistic conversation is about which components matter most and what a sustainable version looks like, which is a conversation most patients have never been offered.

11.6 Infection Control on the Ward

Bronchiectasis carries an infection control dimension that general wards handle inconsistently, and the inconsistency causes real distress to patients who understand the issue better than the staff caring for them.

Patients with chronic colonisation, particularly with organisms that are difficult to eradicate, are at risk of cross infection from other patients with suppurative lung disease. Segregation practice is well established in cystic fibrosis services and applied patchily elsewhere. The practical implication on an acute ward is that two patients with bronchiectasis should not routinely share a bay, and that a patient who tells you they should not be near another chest patient is usually right and has usually been told so by their specialist team.

Sputum pots need lids, disposal needs to be prompt, and clearance sessions generate aerosol. A patient performing 20 minutes of huffing in an open bay is doing exactly what they have been asked to do in exactly the wrong place.

Offering a side room or a screened area for clearance is a small provision that patients notice.

Hand hygiene after handling sputum pots is obvious and is the step most often compressed on a busy round. Nebuliser equipment requires cleaning and drying between uses according to local policy, and a nebuliser chamber left damp on a bedside locker becomes its own reservoir.

None of this requires specialist knowledge. It requires somebody to notice that a patient with a chronically infected airway has been placed opposite another one.

11.7 Recognising the Exacerbation

The following is a composite case; identifying details have been changed.

Background

Tierney, aged 66, had bronchiectasis diagnosed nine years earlier, with chronic colonisation identified on previous sampling. She had been admitted twice in the preceding year and was under a respiratory service.

Presentation

She was admitted from the emergency department with breathlessness and fever. Her sputum was recorded as green on the admission clerking. She was commenced on standard community acquired pneumonia treatment.

Analysis

Green sputum was Tierney's baseline and had been for years, which was documented in her respiratory clinic letters and not in her admission notes. The finding that identified the exacerbation was a different one. Her daily volume had approximately doubled over four days, her clearance sessions had become ineffective, and she had experienced increasing fatigue for a week before any fever appeared. Her prior sampling results, which were available, indicated an organism unlikely to respond to the antibiotic she had been given.

Intervention

The respiratory team was contacted, previous sampling results were retrieved, and antibiotic therapy was changed. A physiotherapy referral was made for clearance during the admission, and nebulised saline was reinstated, having been omitted on admission because it was not on her general practice repeat list.

Outcome

She improved over six days and was discharged. Her clearance regimen at discharge was simplified at her request from twice daily to once daily with an agreed plan to increase during exacerbations, a compromise the physiotherapist described as clinically imperfect and more likely to be followed than the previous prescription had been.

Teaching Points

Sputum colour without a baseline is not a clinical finding. Volume change and clearance effectiveness carried the diagnostic information here.

Previous microbiology in a patient with established colonisation should be retrieved before empirical treatment is chosen rather than after it fails.

Regular nebulised therapies are frequently omitted on admission because they do not appear on a repeat prescription list, and reinstating them is a nursing task nobody is formally allocated.

Bringing It Together

The practical position is that four things determine whether a patient with bronchiectasis does well, and three of them are nursing tasks.

Ask the patient to describe their morning in sequence. Bronchodilator, then hyperosmolar agent, then clearance, then inhaled antibiotic. Sequence errors are common, invisible on a chart, and correctable in one conversation.

Establish the sputum baseline and record it somewhere the next admitting team will find it. Volume, colour, and viscosity when well. Without it, the most useful monitoring data the patient generates is uninterpretable, and Tierney's case shows what happens when the admitting team has to guess.

Watch the huff. It is the single most commonly mistaught component of clearance and the difference between a huff and a cough is visible and audible in one demonstration.

And be realistic about the burden. A regimen the patient will actually perform once daily beats a regimen they abandon after a fortnight, and negotiating that trade off openly is better clinical practice than prescribing an ideal and recording non adherence when it does not happen.

The fourth thing, the microbiology, belongs to the medical team, and the nursing contribution to it is to ensure a decent sample is sent before the first dose of antibiotic rather than after. Retrieve the previous results too. A patient with nine years of documented colonisation has a microbiological history that predicts the current organism better than any empirical guess, and it sits in a clinic letter that takes two minutes to find.

One further point applies to every patient in this chapter. Pulmonary rehabilitation is recommended for people with bronchiectasis who have impaired exercise tolerance (Hill et al., 2019), and it is offered to this group far less often than to patients with obstructive disease. A patient who is breathless on exertion and has never been referred is a referral waiting to be made, and it can be made from a ward.

Chapter 11 Review Questions

1. In what order should a patient with bronchiectasis perform bronchodilator, nebulised hypertonic saline, airway clearance, and inhaled antibiotic?

A) Clearance, bronchodilator, hypertonic saline, inhaled antibiotic

B) Bronchodilator, hypertonic saline, clearance, inhaled antibiotic

C) Hypertonic saline, clearance, bronchodilator, inhaled antibiotic

D) Inhaled antibiotic, bronchodilator, hypertonic saline, clearance

Answer: B. The bronchodilator opens the airway and reduces bronchospasm provoked by hypertonic saline. The hyperosmolar agent mobilises secretions before clearance. The inhaled antibiotic is delivered last into a cleared airway.

2. A patient with bronchiectasis produces green sputum on admission. What additional information is required before this is interpreted as an exacerbation?

A) The result of a chest radiograph

B) The patient's usual baseline sputum colour and volume

C) The white cell count

D) The date of the last respiratory clinic appointment

Answer: B. Many patients with bronchiectasis produce purulent sputum at baseline. Change from that individual baseline, particularly in volume and clearance effectiveness, carries the information.

3. Why is a forced expiration, or huff, preferred over coughing during airway clearance?

A) It is less tiring and avoids the raised intrathoracic pressure and airway collapse associated with repeated coughing

B) It delivers nebulised drug more effectively

C) It is the only technique validated in bronchiectasis

D) It reduces the need for postural drainage

Answer: A. The huff is a forced exhalation with an open glottis. Patients who convert it into a cough clear less and tire more quickly.

Chapter 12: Interstitial Lung Disease Nursing

Chapter Complexity Level: Advanced

Prerequisites: Chapters 1, 2, and 13 is a useful companion.

Time Investment: One hour to read. One information sheet to build.

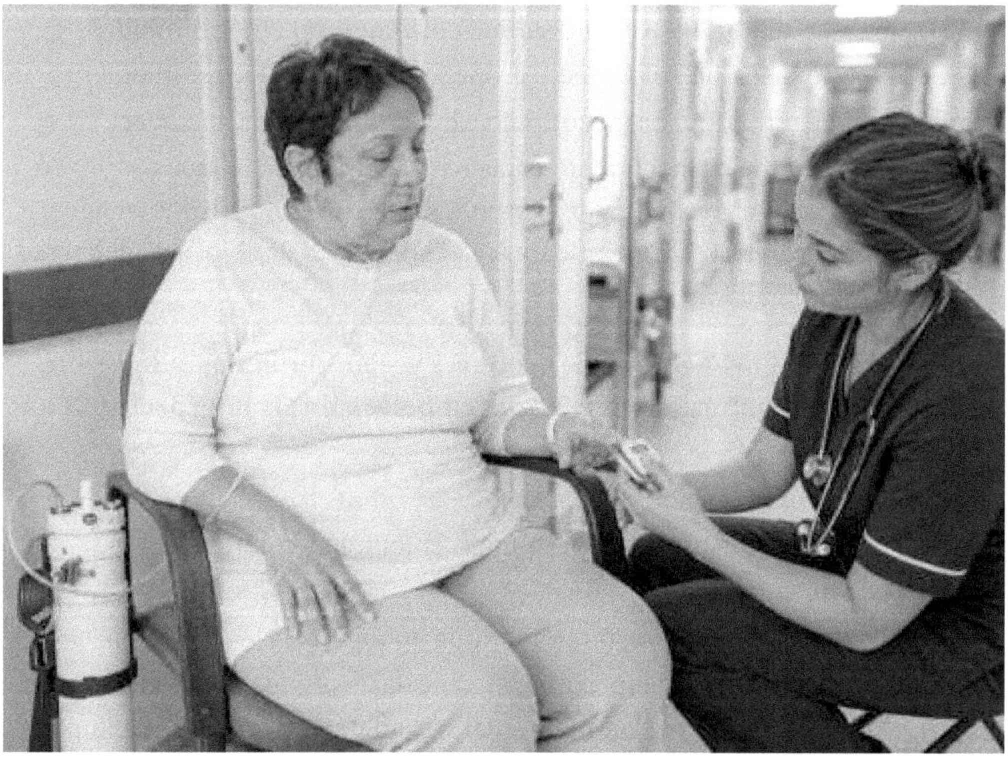

Why does a patient with interstitial lung disease desaturate to 84 percent walking to the toilet while sitting comfortably at 95 percent, when a patient with equally severe chronic obstructive disease often does the reverse? The answer is not a curiosity. It determines how oxygen is assessed in this group, why exercise testing matters more than resting measurement, and why a nurse who checks saturations at the bedside and records them as satisfactory has measured the one situation in which this patient is least impaired. Interstitial disease behaves unlike obstructive disease in ways that make a good deal of standard respiratory nursing subtly wrong.

12.1 What Makes It Different

Interstitial lung disease is a group of conditions in which the tissue between and around the alveoli becomes inflamed, scarred, or both. The airways are not the primary problem. The lung becomes stiff rather than obstructed, and gas transfer across the thickened interface becomes the limiting step.

Three consequences follow and each one changes nursing practice.

Lung volumes fall rather than airflow. Spirometry shows a restrictive pattern, and the useful measurement for monitoring progression is forced vital capacity rather than the measures that dominate obstructive disease.

Gas transfer fails before oxygenation does at rest. At rest, the blood spends long enough in the pulmonary capillary to equilibrate even across a thickened barrier. On exertion, transit time shortens, and equilibration fails. This is why exertional desaturation is the characteristic finding and why resting saturations mislead.

And breathlessness is disproportionate to what the resting numbers suggest. A patient with a resting saturation of 95 percent who cannot cross a room is not exaggerating, and being told that their oxygen levels are fine is a common and damaging experience for this group.

12.2 The Specialist Who Is Not There

Most guidance on interstitial disease assumes a specialist nurse. The service reality does not support that assumption.

A United Kingdom national survey of 122 patient and carer respondents found that only 39 percent of patients had frequent contact with a specialist nurse for this condition, that 36 percent had no access at all, and that only eight trusts routinely allocated a named specialist nurse within six months of diagnosis (Russell et al., 2018). Patient organisations have reported that the specialist nurse is regarded by patients as the single most valuable point of contact for their care.

The practical implication is that a ward nurse, a community matron, or a practice nurse is frequently the entire nursing provision this patient receives. That is the assumption this chapter is written on.

12.3 Oxygen Assessed Properly

Resting oximetry is close to useless as a sole assessment in this population, and it is what most patients receive.

Ambulatory assessment is the relevant measurement. The patient walks, usually a defined distance or for a defined time, with continuous oximetry, and the question is whether they desaturate and by how much. A patient who drops substantially on exertion may benefit from ambulatory oxygen even when their resting saturation is comfortable, and the assessment is what generates the referral.

Two nursing observations feed directly into this. Record what the patient can do, in specific terms, rather than describing exercise tolerance in general adjectives. Kitchen to bathroom. Fourteen stairs with one rest. Those descriptions are reproducible between shifts and between admissions in a way that moderately reduced is not.

And take a saturation after walking rather than only at rest. This takes 90 seconds and is not routine anywhere the author has worked. It frequently produces the finding that generates the referral.

One caution belongs alongside this. Ambulatory oxygen is assessed and prescribed by a specialist service, and a nurse who identifies exertional desaturation has generated a referral rather than a prescription. Long term oxygen therapy is a separate assessment with separate criteria, and the two are frequently confused by patients and by staff.

> **Teaching Point:** *A resting saturation in interstitial disease describes the patient's best moment of the day. Recording it as their oxygenation, without any exertional measurement, systematically understates the problem, and it is the commonest reason ambulatory oxygen assessment is never requested.*

12.4 Antifibrotic Therapy and Why Patients Stop

Antifibrotic drugs slow the rate of decline in lung function in progressive fibrotic disease. They do not improve symptoms, they do not reverse damage, and they have side effects that patients feel every day in exchange for a benefit they cannot perceive at all. That asymmetry explains most discontinuation, and it is the single area where nursing input has the largest effect.

Gastrointestinal effects dominate. Nausea, appetite loss, diarrhoea, and weight loss are common. Photosensitivity and rash occur with one agent and are frequently severe enough to keep patients indoors in summer. Liver function requires monitoring. Fatigue is near universal and is the effect patients rank as most limiting and clinicians record least often.

Practical mitigation is unglamorous and it works. Taking doses with food rather than on an empty stomach. Dividing doses where the regimen permits. Antiemetics and antidiarrhoeals used proactively rather than after a bad week. High factor sun protection and clothing advice given at the point of prescribing rather than after the first burn. Dose reduction, which is a prescriber decision, is very often preferable to discontinuation and patients rarely know it is an option.

The question that surfaces most of this takes ten seconds. Ask what the tablets are doing to them, rather than whether they are taking them. Patients under report side effects to clinicians they believe are invested in the treatment, and a nurse who asks about the burden rather than the adherence gets a different answer.

12.5 Cough, Fatigue, and the Things Nobody Treats

Chronic cough in fibrotic lung disease is under recognised and under treated. It disrupts sleep, causes incontinence and rib pain, and is socially isolating because it is loud and public and frequently assumed by strangers to be infectious.

Reversible contributors should be addressed before the cough is accepted as intrinsic. Reflux is common in this population. Some medications provoke cough. Where the cough remains refractory, options are limited, and speech and language therapy delivered cough suppression techniques have a genuine place that few patients are offered.

Anxiety and depression are common in this group, alongside adjustment difficulty and existential distress relating to a progressive life limiting diagnosis. Psychological distress is identified in the specialist nursing literature as one of the core symptom domains requiring active management, together with breathlessness, fatigue and cough (Russell et al., 2018). Those are not incidental findings and they are not adequately captured by asking a patient whether they are coping. Screening tools exist, they take minutes, and a referral pathway is more useful to the patient than a sympathetic conversation.

Nutrition deserves specific attention because it is frequently missed. Weight loss and muscle wasting are common in advancing fibrotic disease, and pulmonary cachexia carries adverse prognostic weight. Adequate protein intake supports respiratory muscle function and underpins any benefit from pulmonary rehabilitation, which means a dietetic referral is not a comfort measure in this group. A patient who has lost weight steadily across two admissions, with nobody weighing them at either, is a common finding and an easily corrected one.

12.6 The Acute Exacerbation

Patients with fibrotic disease are admitted acutely, and the admission carries a specific trap.

An acute exacerbation of fibrotic interstitial disease is a sudden deterioration in breathlessness and oxygenation without an identified alternative cause. It carries high mortality. It looks, on a general ward at midnight, almost exactly like an infective exacerbation or pulmonary oedema, and it is frequently treated as both while investigations proceed.

The nursing consequence is that oxygen requirements in these patients can escalate very rapidly, over hours rather than days, and a patient stable on nasal cannulae in the evening may need substantially more by morning. Monitoring intervals set on the assumption of an obstructive exacerbation are frequently too widely spaced.

There is a second point that matters more. Noninvasive ventilation and invasive ventilation have a far weaker role here than in the hypercapnic obstructive disease covered in Part III. Outcomes for mechanical ventilation in acute exacerbations of pulmonary fibrosis are poor, which makes the ceiling of care conversation described in Chapter 10 more urgent in this population and not less. A patient with progressive fibrotic disease admitted acutely should have an escalation plan documented early in the admission, and asking whether one exists is a legitimate nursing question on the first ward round rather than the third.

Sitting the patient upright, controlling the environment, and using the airflow and positioning interventions in Chapter 13 will do more for their distress in the first hour than most of the alternatives available on a general ward.

12.7 Two Diagnoses, Two Conversations

The following are composite cases.

Case A

Fable, aged 70, was diagnosed following investigation for breathlessness. At the diagnostic appointment the consultant explained the condition and the treatment. The nurse present asked Fable afterwards what he had understood, and he said that he had a scarring condition and that the tablets would clear it up over a year or so. She corrected that gently at that appointment and again by telephone the following week. When his function declined 14 months later, the conversation about advance care planning built on an understanding that had been developing since the beginning.

Case B

Zennor, aged 68, received the same diagnosis and the same explanation from a different clinician. Nobody checked what she had understood. She interpreted the antifibrotic prescription as treatment intended to cure, told her family so, and stopped it after four months because it was making her feel unwell and not working. She re presented 11 months later with substantially reduced function and no advance planning in place, and the first conversation about prognosis took place during an acute admission.

The diagnosis, the drug, and the information delivered were the same. What differed was whether anyone established what had been heard, which is a nursing act and takes one question.

12.8 Talking About Prognosis Without Owning It

The following account is a composite, with details changed for anonymity.

Xael worked on a respiratory ward and had been asked twice in one week how long a patient had left. Neither patient was under his care in any formal sense. Both had asked him at night, and both had asked him rather than the consultant, which he initially interpreted as a failure of medical communication.

He came to think it was something else. Patients ask the person who is present and who is not going to leave the room in four minutes. The question is frequently not a request for a number.

What he settled on was a sequence. He would ask what had prompted the question. He would answer the part he could answer honestly, which was usually that the condition was progressive, that he could see they were more breathless than at the last admission, and that he did not know how long. He would then ask what they were most worried about, which nearly always produced something concrete and addressable, such as being breathless at the end or being alone or a spouse being unable to cope.

The part he never resolved was the handover. Overnight conversations of this kind rarely survive into daytime planning unless someone deliberately carries them, and Xael's unit had no mechanism for that beyond his own notes. He described writing them up in detail and having no confidence that anyone read them, which is an accurate description of most nursing documentation of conversations.

Teaching points:

The question about prognosis is usually a route into a specific fear, and asking what is worrying them most converts an unanswerable question into an actionable one.

Answering honestly does not require knowing the prognosis. Naming what you can see, and what you do not know, is a complete answer.

The Larger Picture

Interstitial disease inverts several assumptions carried over from obstructive disease. Resting saturations understate impairment rather than reflecting it. The treatment slows decline without relieving symptoms, which makes side effect management the determinant of whether it continues. The most limiting symptoms, cough and fatigue, are the ones least likely to appear in a clinic letter. And the specialist nurse the guidance assumes is absent for more than a third of these patients.

What follows for a ward nurse is a small set of actions that require no specialist training. Walk the patient and record the saturation afterwards. Ask what the tablets are doing to them. Ask what they understood the diagnosis to mean. Screen for anxiety and low mood.

Weigh them, and refer to pulmonary rehabilitation, which benefits this group and is offered to them less often than to patients with obstructive disease.

Those actions share a structure. Each one converts a symptom the patient is carrying privately into a recorded clinical finding that somebody else can act on, and in a population where specialist follow up is unreliable, the recording is the intervention. None of them requires permission, a referral pathway, or a competency sign off, which is fortunate, because for more than a third of these patients there is no specialist nurse to defer to.

They also lead somewhere this chapter has deliberately not gone. Breathlessness in fibrotic disease is frequently refractory, it is frequently present when oxygen is not indicated, and the interventions that help most are not pharmacological. That subject is large enough to need its own treatment, and it applies as much to advanced obstructive disease and heart failure as it does here. Chapter 13 takes it up.

Chapter 12 Review Questions

1. A patient with fibrotic interstitial lung disease has a resting saturation of 95 percent but reports being unable to cross a room. What is the most appropriate nursing action?

A) Reassure the patient that their oxygen levels are satisfactory

B) Record the saturation and review at the next observation round

C) Measure saturation during and after walking, and record specific functional limits

D) Request an urgent arterial blood gas

Answer: C. Exertional desaturation is characteristic of this group because reduced capillary transit time on exertion prevents equilibration across a thickened interface. Resting measurement describes the patient's least impaired state.

2. Why do patients frequently discontinue antifibrotic therapy?

A) The drugs relieve symptoms and are stopped once patients feel better

B) The side effects are experienced daily while the benefit, slowed decline, is not perceptible

C) The drugs require weekly hospital attendance

D) The treatment is only licensed for six months

Answer: B. The asymmetry between felt burden and imperceptible benefit drives discontinuation. Dose reduction is frequently preferable to stopping and patients are often unaware it is an option.

3. What proportion of surveyed patients with interstitial lung disease reported having no access to a specialist nurse?

A) Around 5 percent

B) Around 15 percent

C) Around 36 percent

D) Around 60 percent

Answer: C. In a national survey of 122 patient and carer respondents, 36 percent reported no access at all and only 39 percent had frequent contact, which is why this chapter is written for the generalist.

PART V: BREATHLESSNESS AS A SYMPTOM

Chapter 13: Chronic Breathlessness Beyond Oxygen

Chapter Complexity Level: Intermediate

Prerequisites: Chapters 2 and 12.

Time Investment: One hour to read. One fan intervention to deliver.

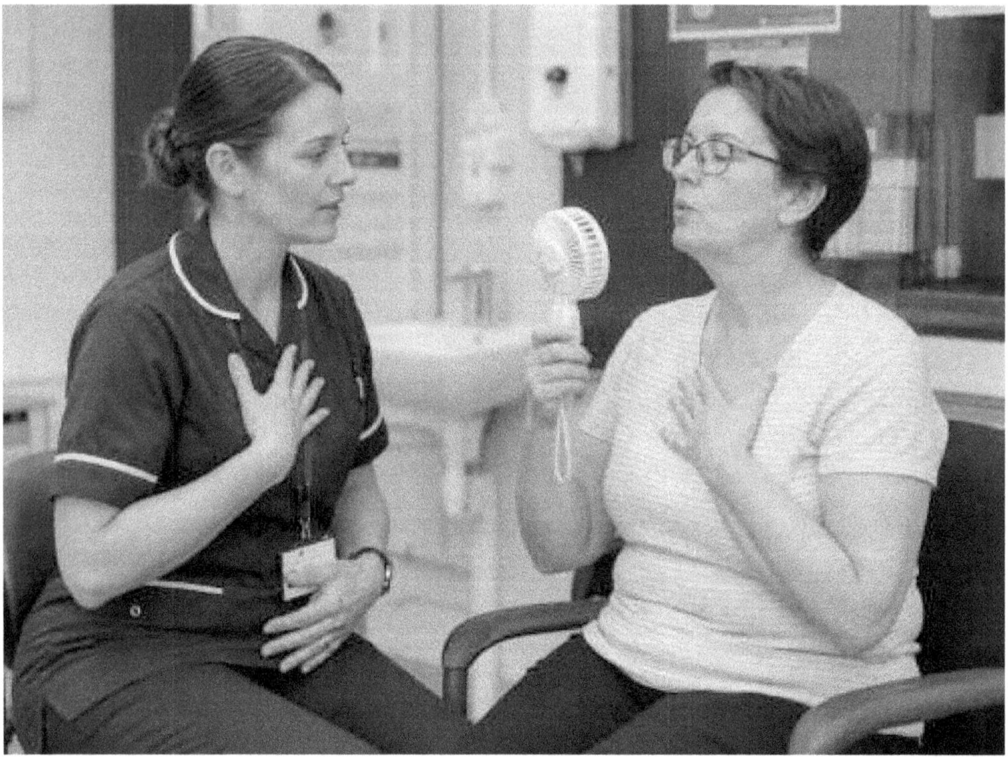

Oxygen is the treatment most requested by breathless patients and most given by clinicians. Oxygen does not relieve breathlessness in patients who are not hypoxaemic. Both of these statements have been supported by evidence for years, and they coexist on every respiratory ward in the country. The gap between them is not explained by ignorance, because most nurses know the second statement is true. It is explained by the fact that a breathless, frightened patient in front of you generates an urgent need to do something, and oxygen is the something that is closest to hand.

13.1 The Problem Stated Concretely

Chronic breathlessness is breathlessness that persists despite optimal treatment of the underlying condition. It is not a failure to diagnose. It is what remains after the diagnosis has been made and treated properly.

Its intensity is not reliably predicted by the severity of the underlying lung pathology (Spathis et al., 2017). Two patients with similar lung function can be differently disabled, and the difference is not explained by the lungs.

That single finding is the reason this chapter exists. If breathlessness tracked lung damage, the only available treatment would be treating the lung damage. Because it does not, there is a substantial component that is modifiable by other means, and those means are largely nursing and allied health interventions rather than prescriptions.

The scale is considerable. Breathlessness affects more than a quarter of community dwelling older adults and most people with chronic respiratory conditions (Spathis et al., 2021). It drives emergency attendance, it causes patients to withdraw from activity, and it frightens families.

13.2 What Has Been Tried

The dominant historical approach was to treat the lung and expect the symptom to follow. Where it did not, the residual breathlessness was frequently attributed to anxiety, deconditioning, or the patient's own management of their condition.

Oxygen filled the gap, and the belief behind it persists among clinicians. In a survey of health professionals attending a three day chronic breathlessness workshop, almost 30 percent indicated that supplemental oxygen for non hypoxaemic patients was an effective strategy for relieving chronic breathlessness (Johnston et al., 2020). Oxygen is available, it is visible, it satisfies the expectation that something has been done, and in hypoxaemic patients it is entirely appropriate. In non hypoxaemic patients it delivers little, and it carries costs that are rarely counted. It tethers people to equipment, it is noisy, it dries the airway, and it establishes a belief that the symptom is an oxygen problem, which makes every subsequent non pharmacological intervention harder to introduce.

The second thing that was tried was advice, and specifically advice to rest. Well intentioned guidance to avoid provoking breathlessness produces reduced activity, which produces deconditioning, which produces more breathlessness at lower workloads. Families compound this by taking over tasks the patient could still perform. The result is a cycle that is driven entirely by reasonable behaviour.

Clinical training has also worked against progress here. Training prioritises disease modification over symptom control, and prescribing is a culturally acceptable and relatively quick action compared with the time and coordinated teamwork that non pharmacological therapies require (Spathis et al., 2017).

13.3 The Model That Changed the Approach

The Breathing, Thinking, Functioning model, proposed by Spathis and colleagues in 2017, reorganised this territory into three cycles that maintain and worsen the symptom, each with its own interventions.

The **breathing** cycle describes the mechanics. Breathlessness produces rapid, shallow, inefficient breathing with accessory muscle use and, in obstructive disease, dynamic hyperinflation. Inefficient breathing increases the work of breathing, which increases breathlessness.

The **thinking** cycle describes the cognitive and emotional response. Attention to the sensation, memories of previous frightening episodes, and catastrophic interpretation produce anxiety and heightened arousal, which amplify the perception of breathlessness.

The **functioning** cycle describes behaviour. Reduced activity leads to deconditioning and to increased reliance on others, which produces more breathlessness on less exertion.

The model's value is practical rather than theoretical. It tells a clinician which intervention to reach for, because each cycle has different treatments, and it gives the patient a rationale. Patients accept a handheld fan more readily when they understand what it is doing than when it is handed to them without explanation.

> **Teaching Point:** *Explaining why an intervention should work is not preamble to the intervention. In breathlessness management it is part of the intervention, because a patient who does not believe a fan will help will not use it during an episode, which is the only time it matters.*

13.4 Airflow and the Handheld Fan

The best evidenced non pharmacological intervention for chronic breathlessness costs a few pounds.

In a randomised controlled crossover trial, 50 participants with advanced disease used a handheld fan directed either at the face or at the leg for five minutes. Breathlessness was significantly reduced when the fan was directed at the face compared with the leg (Galbraith et al., 2010). The mechanism is thought to involve stimulation of facial and nasopharyngeal receptors supplied by the trigeminal nerve, which modifies the central perception of breathlessness.

Two details determine whether it works in practice.

Direction matters. The airflow must be directed at the central face, across the nose and mouth. A fan pointed at the chest or blowing generally around the room is not the intervention that was tested.

Timing matters more. The fan is for use during breathlessness and during recovery from exertion, not as ambient background. Patients need to be told to keep it within reach, to use it at the moment of breathlessness, and to continue for a few minutes after activity has stopped.

An open window and a cool room work by the same mechanism and are free. A patient sitting in an overheated side room with the window closed is in an environment that is actively worsening the symptom.

13.5 Breathing, Pacing, and Rehabilitation

Breathing control means relaxed breathing using the lower chest with the shoulders and upper chest relaxed. It is taught in a settled state and practised before it is needed, because nobody learns a new breathing pattern for the first time during a panic.

Pursed lip breathing has a specific role in obstructive disease. Exhaling against partly closed lips generates back pressure that splints the airways during expiration, reduces air trapping, and slows the respiratory rate. Many patients discover it independently, which is worth telling them, because it validates something they may have been doing apologetically.

The recovery position for breathlessness, leaning forward with the arms supported on a table or on the thighs, fixes the shoulder girdle and allows the accessory muscles to act on the chest wall. This is the tripod position described in Chapter 1 as a sign of distress. It is also a treatment, and patients should be taught to adopt it deliberately.

Pacing is the intervention that addresses the functioning cycle, and it needs care in how it is framed. Pacing is not doing less. It is distributing effort so that more gets done overall, and the distinction matters because patients who understand pacing as restriction abandon it.

Pulmonary rehabilitation is the most effective intervention in this chapter and the one most frequently declined (Bolton et al., 2013). Referral succeeds more often when the patient understands that supervised breathlessness during exercise is safe and intended, because the commonest reason for refusal is a belief that becoming breathless is dangerous. Nurse led breathlessness clinics that combine education with psychological support have shown improvement in breathlessness, performance status, and emotional state, which indicates that the package rather than any single component is what works.

13.6 The Carer Nobody Trained

Carers are the people managing most breathlessness episodes and they receive almost no preparation.

They live with uncertainty about what an episode means, they lack strategies for relieving it, and fear of breathlessness drives demand for emergency healthcare, some of which is avoidable. A carer who has watched somebody struggle to breathe and has been given no instruction will call an ambulance, correctly, because that is the only tool they have been issued.

Teaching the carer takes ten minutes and covers four things. What to do first, which is to open a window or use the fan and help the person into a forward leaning position. How to speak, which is slowly and briefly, because a frightened person cannot process complex sentences. What is expected and what is not. And when to call for help, defined specifically rather than left to judgment.

That last item is what makes the rest safe. A carer given techniques without clear escalation criteria has been handed responsibility without authority.

Carers also need permission to look after themselves, which they rarely take. Sleep is frequently broken for years, and a carer who is exhausted manages episodes less well and becomes unwell themselves. Asking the carer directly how they are sleeping, in front of the patient, legitimises a subject most families do not raise.

13.7 The Patient Who Was Given Oxygen

The following is a composite case; identifying details have been changed.

Background

Hollis, aged 76, had moderate chronic obstructive pulmonary disease and had been admitted four times in a year with breathlessness. On each admission he improved within 48 hours without any change in treatment. His resting saturations were consistently 94 to 96 percent on air.

Presentation

He presented acutely breathless, frightened, with a respiratory rate of 28 and saturations of 95 percent on air. Oxygen was commenced in the emergency department. He settled over the following two hours and the oxygen was recorded as effective.

Analysis

He was not hypoxaemic at any point, which means the oxygen was not correcting a deficit. What had settled him was more likely the combination of time, the presence of staff, and the reduction in fear that arrival at a hospital produces. He had been taught, across four admissions, that oxygen was what relieved his breathlessness, and he had begun requesting it at home.

Intervention

On this admission the respiratory nurse introduced the Breathing, Thinking, Functioning framework in plain terms, provided a handheld fan and taught its use during an episode, taught the forward leaning position and pursed lip breathing, and referred him to pulmonary rehabilitation. His wife was included in all of it.

Outcome

He attended six of 12 rehabilitation sessions and stopped, citing transport difficulty. At six months he had had one further admission rather than four. He continued to use the fan and reported that it helped, though he still described oxygen as the thing that worked, which had not shifted.

Teaching Points

An intervention given during spontaneous recovery will be credited with the recovery, and repeated admissions can teach a patient a causal belief that is difficult to undo.

Partial uptake is the normal outcome. Six sessions attended and a fan used daily is a real result, and recording it as non completion misdescribes it.

13.8 The Conversation That Failed First

The following account is a composite, with details changed for anonymity.

Fallon was a community respiratory nurse who had introduced the handheld fan to her caseload and found that most patients did not use it.

Her initial approach was to hand the fan over with an explanation of the evidence. Patients were polite about it. The fans ended up in drawers.

What changed the uptake was doing it in the wrong order deliberately. Instead of explaining and then demonstrating, she began asking the patient to walk until they became breathless, and then used the fan on them while they recovered. Patients felt the difference themselves before any explanation was offered, and the explanation then landed on an experience rather than on a claim.

She was candid that this does not always work. Some patients felt no benefit, and she stopped presenting the fan as reliably effective. A minority found the sensation unpleasant. She also noted that the demonstration requires the patient to become breathless in front of you, which some find humiliating, and that asking permission first mattered more than she had expected.

Teaching points:

An intervention demonstrated during recovery from exertion is experienced rather than described, and uptake follows experience.

Not every patient benefits, and presenting the fan as universally effective damages credibility for the interventions that follow.

What Earns Its Place

Hollis still says that oxygen is the thing that works. Four admissions taught him that, and one admission with a fan and a rehabilitation referral did not undo it. He also had one admission in the following six months instead of four, and he uses the fan every day. Both of those things are true about the same man, and a chapter that reported only the second would be selling something.

What earns its place in practice is the small set of interventions that are cheap, evidenced, and deliverable by a nurse without a prescription. Airflow to the face during an episode. The forward leaning position, taught deliberately rather than observed as a sign of distress. Pursed lip breathing in obstructive disease. A rationale the patient can repeat back, because belief determines use. Pacing framed as doing more rather than less. A referral to pulmonary rehabilitation with the fear of breathlessness addressed directly, because that fear is the usual reason for refusal. And ten minutes with the carer, including explicit escalation criteria.

What does not earn its place is oxygen for a patient who is not hypoxaemic. It is not neutral, it is not merely ineffective, and every time it is given during a spontaneous recovery it teaches the patient something that will be difficult to unteach later.

The harder truth underneath this chapter is that none of these interventions is difficult, expensive, or new. The 2010 fan trial is old enough to have been in practice for over a decade. What has been missing is not evidence.

Chapter 13 Review Questions

1. **A patient with advanced COPD is breathless at rest with saturations of 95 percent on air. What is the most appropriate first intervention?**

A) Commence oxygen at 2 litres via nasal cannulae

B) Direct airflow across the face, assist into a forward leaning position, and stay with the patient

C) Request an urgent arterial blood gas

D) Advise the patient to rest until the episode passes

Answer: B. The patient is not hypoxaemic, so oxygen has no deficit to correct. Facial airflow, positioning, and presence address the breathing and thinking cycles. Option D contributes to the deconditioning described in section 13.2.

2. **In the trial evidence for the handheld fan, what was the comparison that demonstrated benefit?**

A) Fan against no intervention

B) Fan directed at the face against fan directed at the leg

C) Fan against low flow oxygen

D) Fan against breathing control exercises

Answer: B. Participants crossed over between facial and leg airflow, and breathlessness was significantly reduced with facial airflow. This is why direction of airflow matters when teaching the technique.

3. **Which statement best describes pacing as an intervention?**

A) Reducing overall activity to avoid provoking breathlessness

B) Distributing effort across a day so that more is achieved overall

C) Increasing exercise intensity progressively under supervision

D) Delegating physically demanding tasks to a carer

Answer: B. Framing pacing as restriction leads patients to abandon it, and option A describes the behaviour that generates the deconditioning cycle the intervention is meant to interrupt.

Chapter 14: Breathlessness at Life's End

Chapter Complexity Level: Advanced

Prerequisites: Chapters 10 and 13.

Time Investment: One hour to read. Three responses to rehearse aloud.

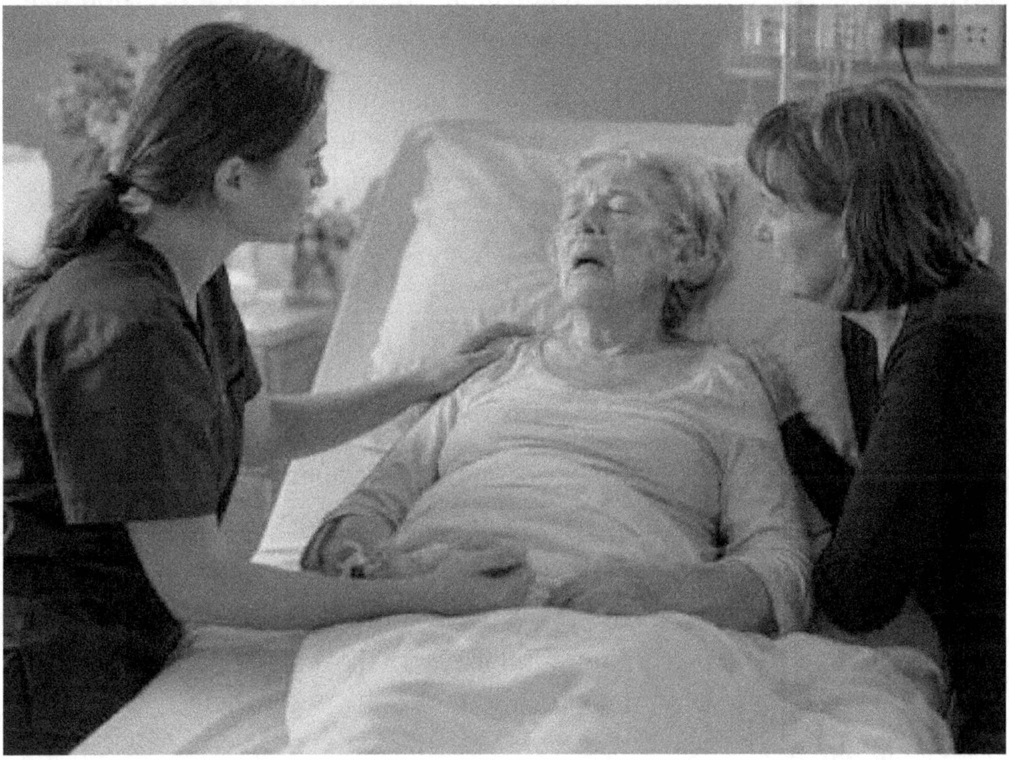

The daughter was standing in the corridor because she could not be in the room. Inside, her father was propped at forty five degrees, breathing at thirty two, eyes open, hands gripping the blanket. A healthcare assistant had put the oxygen back on twice and he had pulled it off twice. The night nurse had been in three times in forty minutes and had said, each time, that the doctor had been bleeped. It was ten past four. The daughter asked the question that nobody on the ward that night had a prepared answer for, which was whether her father was going to suffocate.

14.1 What Was Actually Happening

Tierney was 83 and had advanced fibrotic lung disease. He had been admitted eight days earlier and had been recognised as dying two days before this night. A do not attempt cardiopulmonary resuscitation decision was documented.

Anticipatory medication had been discussed on the ward round on Friday and had not been prescribed.

It was now Sunday. The patient was distressed, the prescription chart contained nothing that could be given for breathlessness, and the on call doctor was covering four wards. The nurse had bleeped twice. The delay was not anyone's negligence. It was the predictable consequence of a decision that had been made verbally and not converted into a prescription before the weekend.

What the daughter saw was her father fighting for air while staff repeatedly told her that help was coming. What she was not told, because nobody had said it, was that he was dying, that his breathing pattern was expected, and that the plan was to make him comfortable rather than to fix him.

She learned both of those things at twenty to five, from a doctor she had never met, in a corridor.

14.2 The Three Failures

Three things went wrong and only one of them was pharmacological.

Anticipatory prescribing had not happened. Medication for breathlessness, agitation, pain, and secretions should be prescribed at the point a patient is recognised as dying, not at the point the symptom appears. The gap between recognising dying and prescribing for it is where most out of hours distress in this situation is generated, and Friday afternoon is the specific danger point.

The family had not been prepared. Nobody had described what the last hours might look like, which meant every change was interpreted as a crisis and as evidence that something was being done wrong.

And the language had failed. Saying that the doctor has been bleeped is accurate and it communicates that the situation is being escalated, which implies it is being fixed. Repeated three times over forty minutes, it becomes a promise that is not being kept.

> **Teaching Point:** *When a patient is recognised as dying, ask on that ward round whether anticipatory medication has been prescribed and whether the family has been told what to expect. Both questions take ten seconds and both are nursing questions. Neither requires you to be the person who does the prescribing or the explaining.*

14.3 Why This Symptom Frightens

Breathlessness at the end of life is different from other terminal symptoms in one respect that shapes everything about managing it. It frightens the people watching almost as much as the person experiencing it.

Pain is largely invisible. Breathlessness is loud, visible, and instinctively recognisable as a threat. Relatives who have coped with a great deal find that they cannot stay in the room, and they frequently interpret the breathing as suffering even when the patient is not distressed.

The distinction between breathlessness and observed respiratory changes matters here. A dying patient may develop rapid, shallow, or irregular breathing, or noisy breathing from retained secretions, without experiencing distress. Families reliably interpret these as suffering. So, sometimes, do staff, and treatment gets escalated in response to the observers' distress rather than the patient's.

The reverse error also occurs. A patient who is quiet may be exhausted rather than comfortable, and the difference is visible in the face and in the hands.

14.4 Medication and the Conversation About It

Opioids are the mainstay of pharmacological management of breathlessness at the end of life. They reduce the sensation of breathlessness through central mechanisms, and their use for this indication is well established in palliative practice. Benzodiazepines have a place where anxiety is a substantial component, which it frequently is, and they are less useful where the dominant problem is the sensation itself.

Doses, routes, and titration are prescribing decisions and they belong in local palliative care guidance and to the prescriber. What belongs to nursing is everything around them, and that is a larger share of the outcome than it appears.

Monitoring is one part. Respiratory rate, level of distress, and comfort, recorded so that the effect of a dose can actually be judged. A medication given without any recorded assessment before or after cannot be titrated by the next person.

The conversation is the other part, and it is the one that most often determines whether the medication is given at all. Families frequently believe that morphine will hasten death, and a family who believes this will resist it, sometimes in the room, sometimes at three in the morning to a nurse who was not expecting the question.

The honest answer is not a reassurance that morphine is harmless. It is that opioids used at appropriate doses to relieve breathlessness are used to treat a symptom rather than to shorten life, that the aim is comfort, and that a person who is not fighting to breathe is generally more comfortable rather than less alert in any way that matters at this stage. Saying that plainly, and acknowledging that the fear is a common one rather than a foolish one, works better than a clinical explanation of receptor physiology.

Some relatives ask directly whether the drug will be what kills him. Answering with a script fails. Answering with what you actually think, which is that he is dying of his lung disease and that the medicine is for the distress, is both truthful and usually sufficient.

14.5 Oxygen at the Very End

Oxygen in the last hours requires a different judgment from oxygen at any other point in this book.

If the patient is hypoxaemic and the oxygen provides comfort, it continues. If the patient is not hypoxaemic, or if the mask is distressing them, the airflow and positioning interventions in Chapter 13 are more effective and considerably less intrusive.

The difficult version is the patient who repeatedly removes the mask. This is information, and it is frequently overridden. A mask replaced for the third time on a dying patient who keeps taking it off is being applied for the benefit of the observers.

Removing oxygen at the end of life can be the kinder act and it needs explaining before it is done, because families interpret withdrawal as giving up. The framing that works is that the mask is no longer helping him and is getting in the way of being with him, and that a fan and an open window achieve more at this point.

14.6 The Room and the Words

The environment does more than most interventions available in the last hours. Cool air, an open window, a fan directed across the face, reduced noise, dimmed lighting, and an upright or forward leaning position supported with pillows.

Mouth care matters disproportionately. Mouth breathing in the last hours produces severe dryness, and regular mouth care is among the interventions relatives most value and most readily learn to do themselves, which gives them something to do with their hands.

The words matter as much. Short sentences. A frightened, breathless, or dying person cannot process complex speech, and long reassuring explanations are experienced as noise.

For the question the daughter asked in the corridor, an honest answer exists. It is that people do not usually experience the end as suffocating, that the breathing changes as the body slows, that the medication is there specifically to prevent distress, and that somebody will be watching for it. What must not be said is that he is not suffocating when nobody knows what he is experiencing, or that everything is fine.

For the relative who asks how long, the answer is that you do not know, that you can see he is very unwell, and what you are watching for. For the relative who has just left the room and returns to find the breathing changed, the answer is that this is expected and that it does not mean he is in pain.

Rehearse these aloud before you need them. Reading them is not the same as having said them, and the moment they are required is not a moment for composition.

14.7 Two Nights

The following are composite cases.

Case A

Dune was recognised as dying on a Thursday. Anticipatory medication was prescribed that afternoon. The nurse looking after him spent 15 minutes with his son describing what the next days might involve, including the breathing changes and the noisy secretions. When his breathing became rapid on Saturday night, the son recognised what he had been told to expect, and the nurse gave medication that was already prescribed. The son stayed in the room.

Case B

Umber was recognised as dying on a Thursday. The conversation about anticipatory medication took place and the prescription was deferred to the next ward round, which was Monday. When she became distressed on Saturday night her family were told the doctor had been called. She received medication after 90 minutes. Her daughter later said that the ninety minutes was the part she could not stop thinking about.

The clinical trajectories were similar and both patients died comfortably in the end. What differed was one prescription written three days earlier and one conversation held before it was needed. Neither of those is a specialist palliative care intervention. Both are things a ward nurse can ask for on a Thursday.

14.8 The Nurse Who Left the Room

The following account is a composite, with details changed for anonymity.

Vesper had been qualified for two years and described leaving a dying patient's room because she did not know what to say to his wife.

She said afterwards that she had understood the clinical situation perfectly well. What she had not been given, at any point in her training, was any preparation for being the person in the room when somebody is frightened and there is nothing left to fix. Her instinct had been that she needed the right words, could not find them, and therefore should not be there.

What changed her practice was a colleague telling her that presence is the intervention and that silence is permitted. She began staying, saying less, and doing small physical things, mouth care, repositioning a pillow, adjusting the fan, which gave her a reason to remain and gave the family a model to copy.

She was clear that this did not become comfortable. She described still finding it difficult four years later, and said that the difference was that she now stayed while finding it difficult rather than leaving. Her unit had no routine debrief, and she noted that most of what she had learned about this had come from one conversation with one colleague, which is a fragile way for a workforce to acquire a core skill.

Teaching points:

Presence without words is a legitimate and effective intervention, and staff frequently leave because they believe it is not.

Small physical acts of care give both nurse and family a way to remain in the room when speech is not possible.

The Core of It

The daughter in the corridor at ten past four was not asking for a prognosis. She was asking whether her father was suffering, and whether anybody was going to stop it. Those questions had answers available that night. The answers were not given because nobody had prepared her, because the medication that would have addressed the symptom had not been prescribed on Friday, and because the phrase that was offered three times described a process rather than a plan.

None of the three failures required specialist palliative care to prevent. Asking on the ward round whether anticipatory medication is prescribed takes ten seconds. Describing what the last days may look like takes fifteen minutes and can be done by any nurse who has seen it. Replacing the doctor has been bleeped with a description of what is happening and what will be done about it requires only that somebody has thought about the sentence in advance.

That is why this chapter contains scripts rather than principles. Under pressure, at four in the morning, with a frightened relative in a corridor, principles evaporate and sentences survive. The nurses who manage these nights well are not the ones with the best understanding of opioid pharmacology. They are the ones who have said these things before, or rehearsed them, and who have learned that staying in the room while not knowing what to say is itself the thing that helps.

Tierney died at six fifteen, comfortable, after medication was eventually prescribed and given. His daughter was with him. What she remembers is the corridor.

Chapter 14 Review Questions

1. A patient is recognised as dying on a Friday afternoon. Anticipatory medication has been discussed but not prescribed. What is the most appropriate nursing action?

A) Await the next scheduled ward round

B) Request that the prescription is written before the weekend

C) Document the discussion and escalate only if symptoms develop

D) Arrange a specialist palliative care referral instead

Answer: B. The interval between recognising dying and prescribing for it is where avoidable out of hours distress is generated. A prescription written in advance costs nothing if it is not needed.

2. A dying patient repeatedly removes their oxygen mask. What does this most likely indicate?

A) Confusion requiring the mask to be secured

B) That the mask is distressing them and alternatives such as facial airflow should be considered

C) That the oxygen concentration is inadequate

D) That sedation is required

Answer: B. Repeated removal is information. Where the patient is not hypoxaemic, or where the mask itself is the problem, airflow and positioning are more effective and less intrusive.

3. A relative asks whether morphine will hasten their family member's death. Which response is most appropriate?

A) Explain that morphine is entirely harmless

B) Acknowledge that this is a common concern, explain that the medication treats the distress while the underlying illness is what is causing the death, and that the aim is comfort

C) Refer the question to the medical team without responding

D) Explain the receptor mechanism by which opioids reduce breathlessness

Answer: B. The concern is common and reasonable. A plain, honest answer that names the fear works better than reassurance that overstates the case or a technical explanation that does not address what was asked.

PART VI: PROCEDURES AND TRANSITIONS

Chapter 15: Chest Drains and Tracheostomy

Chapter Complexity Level: Advanced

Prerequisites: Chapter 1. Local chest drain and tracheostomy policies.

Time Investment: Ninety minutes to read. One bedside equipment audit.

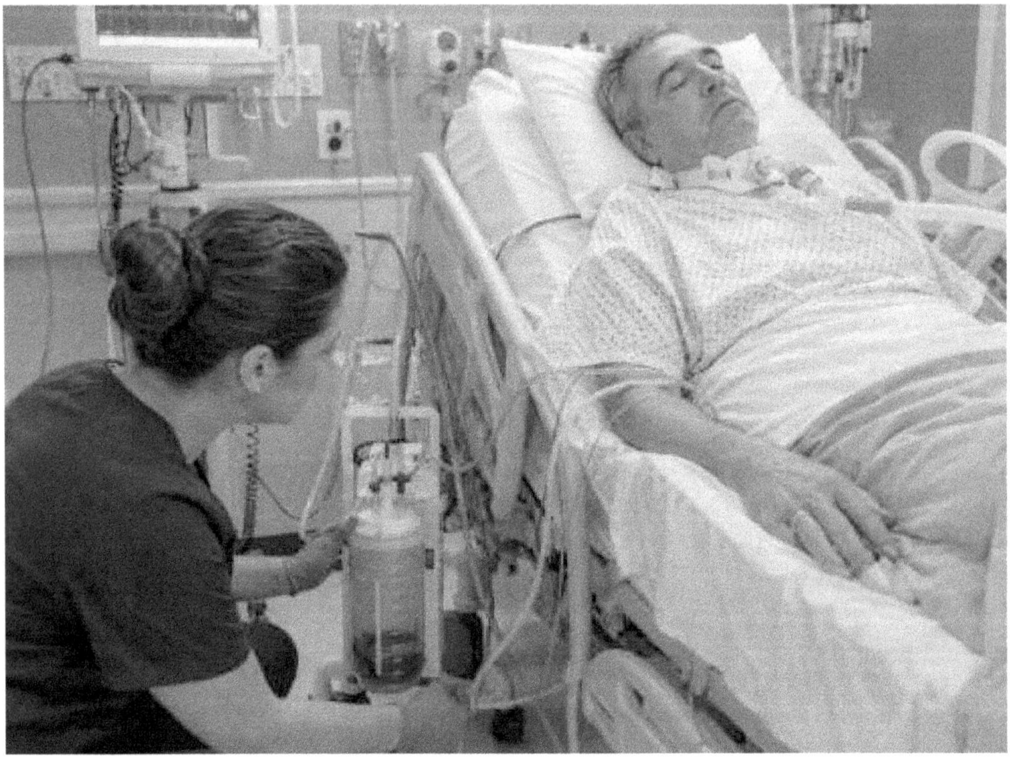

The bottle sits on the floor beside the bed, half hidden by the locker, with a strip of tape marking the fluid level and a date written on it in biro. Most staff walking past it look at the volume in the chamber. The volume is the least informative thing about it. What that bottle reports, minute by minute, is whether air is leaving the pleural space, whether the pleural pressure is changing with respiration, and whether the tube connecting it to the patient is still doing anything at all. Almost all of that information is free, visible from the end of the bed, and routinely unrecorded.

15.1 What the Bottle Reports

An underwater seal drain does three jobs simultaneously and understanding them makes every subsequent observation interpretable. Chest drain and pleural procedure practice in the United Kingdom is governed by the British Thoracic Society pleural disease guideline (Roberts et al., 2023), from which local policy derives.

It allows air or fluid to leave the pleural space. It prevents anything travelling back in, because the tube sits under water and the water acts as a one way valve. And it displays what is happening, through two observable phenomena.

Swinging is the movement of the fluid level in the tube with respiration. Pleural pressure changes with each breath and the fluid column follows it. Swinging tells you the tube is patent and in communication with the pleural space. Its disappearance means either the lung has fully re expanded around the drain or the tube has become blocked or kinked, and those two possibilities have opposite implications.

Bubbling is air passing through the water. It indicates air leaving the pleural space, which is expected in a pneumothorax and expected to reduce as the leak seals. New bubbling in a patient who had stopped bubbling is a new air leak and it is significant.

The chamber must stay below the level of the patient's chest, upright, and never lifted above the insertion site, because raising it can allow fluid to siphon back.

> **Teaching Point:** *Record swinging and bubbling at every observation set, not just drainage volume. A drain that has stopped swinging overnight and is documented only as draining well has had its most important observation omitted.*

15.2 Reading a Drain in Practice

The following worked example uses a composite case.

Joss, aged 44, has a chest drain inserted for a pneumothorax. At the start of the shift the drain is swinging and bubbling intermittently. Four hours later the nurse notes that it is neither swinging nor bubbling, and the patient reports feeling better.

Step one, the two possibilities. Cessation of swinging means either full lung re expansion, which is good and consistent with the patient feeling better, or an obstructed or displaced tube, which is not.

Step two, what distinguishes them. Ask the patient to cough or take a deep breath and watch the fluid column. A patent tube in a re expanded lung usually shows a small movement on coughing. Absolutely no movement on coughing raises the possibility of obstruction. Check the tubing along its whole length for kinks, for dependent loops holding fluid, and for the patient lying on it, which is the commonest cause and the easiest to miss.

Step three, the patient. Assess as in Chapter 1. Respiratory rate, work of breathing, saturations, and whether there is any subcutaneous emphysema, which is the crackling sensation under the skin around the site that indicates air tracking into the tissues.

The complicating moment. Joss's tubing is clear, there is no movement on coughing, and he feels better with normal observations. The obvious conclusion is re expansion. The nurse escalates anyway and requests a chest radiograph, on the grounds that she cannot distinguish the two possibilities at the bedside and that the consequence of being wrong differs enormously between them. The radiograph confirms re expansion. She was right about the outcome and right to escalate, and those are separate judgments.

What this shows. Bedside assessment narrowed the possibilities and could not resolve them. Recognising which observations you cannot interpret is a competence rather than a deficiency, and escalating an ambiguous finding in a patient who feels well is defensible precisely because the alternative diagnosis is dangerous.

15.3 Emergencies and Clamping

Four drain emergencies need an immediate response and the response is not intuitive in three of them.

If the drain becomes disconnected from the tubing, the priority is to re establish a seal. Local policy governs the detail, and the usual immediate action is to place the end of the tube in sterile water to recreate an underwater seal while help is summoned. Never clamp a disconnected drain in a patient with an air leak.

If the drain falls out of the patient, cover the site immediately. Policies vary between an occlusive dressing and a dressing sealed on three sides, and the reason for the debate is the risk of converting an open pneumothorax into a tension pneumothorax by sealing air in. Know what your policy says before you need it, summon urgent help, and observe closely for deterioration.

If the bottle is knocked over, set it upright immediately and check the water level. Most modern systems tolerate this. Escalate and document.

If the patient deteriorates suddenly with a drain in situ, consider tension pneumothorax. Increasing breathlessness, falling saturations, tachycardia, hypotension, and tracheal deviation constitute an emergency requiring immediate senior assistance.

Clamping deserves its own paragraph because it is the intervention most often performed wrongly. Clamping a drain in a patient with an ongoing air leak can produce a tension pneumothorax, which is why routine clamping during transfer or for patient mobility is not appropriate. The narrow legitimate uses, such as clamping briefly when changing a bottle or under specific medical instruction when assessing whether a drain can be removed, are protocol driven and supervised. A drain should never be clamped simply because a patient is going for a scan.

15.4 After a Pleural Procedure

Patients return to the ward after aspiration, drain insertion, and biopsy, and the observation period afterwards is where complications appear.

Pneumothorax following a pleural procedure presents as increasing breathlessness, falling saturations, and chest discomfort, typically within the first hours. Observations should be frequent in that window rather than resumed at the ward's routine interval.

Re expansion pulmonary oedema is uncommon and it is the reason large volume drainage is limited in a single session. It presents as breathlessness, cough, and frothy sputum after a large volume has been removed. Patients who report significant chest discomfort during drainage should have it stopped and reported rather than encouraged to tolerate it.

Bleeding, infection at the site, and pain are the remaining considerations, and pain is the one most often undertreated. A chest drain hurts, particularly on movement and coughing, and inadequate analgesia produces a patient who will not take deep breaths or cough, which produces the sputum retention and atelectasis the drain was partly meant to prevent.

15.5 Tracheostomy on a General Ward

A tracheostomy patient on a general ward is a patient whose airway depends on a tube that ward staff use infrequently, and infrequency is the problem.

Humidification is the first principle and the most neglected. A tracheostomy bypasses the nose, which normally warms and humidifies inspired air. Without humidification, secretions thicken and the tube blocks, and tube blockage is the commonest ward tracheostomy emergency. Humidification is not optional and its interruption for a few hours has consequences.

Inner cannula care is the practical corollary. A tube with an inner cannula allows the inner tube to be removed and cleaned or replaced without disturbing the airway, and regular checking is what prevents an obstruction becoming an emergency.

Suction clears secretions the patient cannot clear themselves and it is performed according to local competency requirements.

Two pieces of information determine safe care and both must be visible at the bedside. Whether the patient has a potentially patent upper airway or is a laryngectomy patient, and what size and type of tube is in place. Those distinctions are the basis of the national bed head signage, and confusing a tracheostomy with a laryngectomy in an emergency is catastrophic, because oxygen delivered to the face of a laryngectomy patient reaches nothing.

Emergency equipment must be present at the bedside at all times, including spare tubes of the same size and one size smaller, a tracheal dilator, suction, and the emergency algorithms. An equipment audit takes two minutes per patient and is the single most useful thing in this section.

Communication is the other daily reality. A patient with a cuffed tube cannot speak. Providing a means of communication is a clinical requirement rather than a courtesy, and speech and language therapy involvement is part of standard multidisciplinary care.

The practical provisions are simple and frequently absent. A pen and paper or a writing board within reach of the hand the patient can actually use. An agreed signal for urgent attention that does not depend on the call bell being reachable. A habit among staff of asking questions that can be answered with a nod or a shake rather than open questions the patient cannot answer. And time, because reading lips or handwriting takes longer than listening and a rushed exchange teaches the patient not to try.

Swallowing is the related concern. A patient with a tracheostomy is at risk of aspiration, and decisions about oral intake belong to a speech and language therapy assessment rather than to a well meaning trial at the bedside. A family bringing in a favourite drink is a common and understandable event, and it needs a conversation rather than a prohibition.

15.6 When the Tube Blocks

The following is a composite case; identifying details have been changed.

Background

Zephyr, aged 61, had a tracheostomy following prolonged ventilation and had been stepped down to a respiratory ward. He was six days into his ward stay, self ventilating, and mobilising short distances.

Presentation

At approximately two in the morning he became acutely distressed, with increased work of breathing, falling saturations, and an inability to make any sound. Suction catheter passage met resistance.

Analysis

Inability to pass a suction catheter in a distressed tracheostomy patient indicates tube obstruction or displacement until proven otherwise. The national algorithms, developed by the National Tracheostomy Safety Project, direct a universal approach beginning with calling for help, applying oxygen to both the face and the stoma, and assessing tube patency (McGrath et al., 2012). Applying oxygen to both sites is the default emergency action for a patient with a tracheostomy, because at that moment it is not always known which route is working.

Intervention

The nurse called for help, applied oxygen to face and stoma, and attempted to remove the inner cannula, which was occluded with thick, dried secretions. Removing it restored ventilation immediately.

Outcome

Zephyr recovered without further intervention. A review established that his heated humidification had been disconnected during a transfer to radiology approximately 14 hours earlier and had not been reconnected on return. The bedside emergency equipment was found to be complete apart from the smaller spare tube.

Teaching Points

Inability to pass a suction catheter in a distressed tracheostomy patient is an emergency finding, not a technical difficulty.

Applying oxygen to both face and stoma is the default first action because the functioning route may not yet be known.

Humidification interrupted during transfer and not reconnected is a recognised and entirely preventable cause of tube obstruction, and checking it on return from any procedure is a nursing task nobody is formally allocated.

Essential Takeaways

The practical position across both halves of this chapter is the same, which is that the safety of these patients rests on observations that take seconds and are routinely omitted.

For chest drains, record swinging and bubbling at every observation set rather than volume alone, and treat the disappearance of swinging as a question rather than as good news. Know your unit's policy on a dislodged drain before you meet one, because the difference between sealing a site fully and sealing it on three sides is a decision nobody should be making from first principles at three in the morning. Do not clamp a drain for transfer. Treat pain properly, because a patient who will not cough acquires a second problem.

For tracheostomy, check humidification, check the bedside equipment, and check the bed head sign, on every shift and after every return from any department. Zephyr's emergency was set in motion 14 hours earlier by a disconnected circuit that nobody looked at, and it was resolved by a nurse who followed a sequence rather than improvising one.

Practise finding the algorithm on your own ward, physically, before you need it. Knowing that it exists is not the same as knowing which wall it is on.

Learn the emergency algorithms before you need them. They exist because these events are uncommon on general wards, which means the staff present will not have managed one recently, which is precisely the circumstance in which a memorised sequence outperforms clinical reasoning.

And be honest about the limits of your own competence with these devices. Suction, inner cannula management, and drain care are all governed by local competency frameworks for good reason. Recognising what you are not signed off to do, and calling early rather than attempting it, is not timidity in this territory. It is the correct clinical judgment.

Chapter 15 Review Questions

1. A chest drain that was swinging and bubbling has stopped doing both overnight. The patient feels better and observations are normal. What is the appropriate interpretation?

A) The lung has re expanded and no action is required

B) The tube is blocked and should be flushed

C) Either re expansion or tube obstruction is possible, and the finding requires assessment and escalation

D) The drain should be clamped and removed

Answer: C. Cessation of swinging has two possible explanations with opposite implications, and they cannot be reliably distinguished at the bedside. Escalating an ambiguous finding is appropriate even when the patient appears well.

2. Why should a chest drain not be clamped routinely for patient transfer?

A) It increases the risk of infection at the insertion site

B) In a patient with an ongoing air leak, clamping can produce a tension pneumothorax

C) It causes the underwater seal to be lost

D) It prevents accurate measurement of drainage volume

Answer: B. Clamping prevents air escaping from the pleural space. Legitimate clamping is protocol driven and supervised, such as during a bottle change.

3. A tracheostomy patient becomes acutely distressed and a suction catheter cannot be passed. What is the immediate action?

A) Attempt to reinsert the tracheostomy tube

B) Call for help and apply oxygen to both the face and the stoma

C) Deflate the cuff and observe

D) Increase the humidification setting

Answer: B. Applying oxygen to both routes is the default emergency action in the national algorithms because the functioning route may not yet be known. Inability to pass a suction catheter indicates obstruction or displacement.

Chapter 16: Discharge That Holds

Chapter Complexity Level: Intermediate

Prerequisites: All preceding chapters.

Time Investment: One hour to read. One discharge document to rewrite.

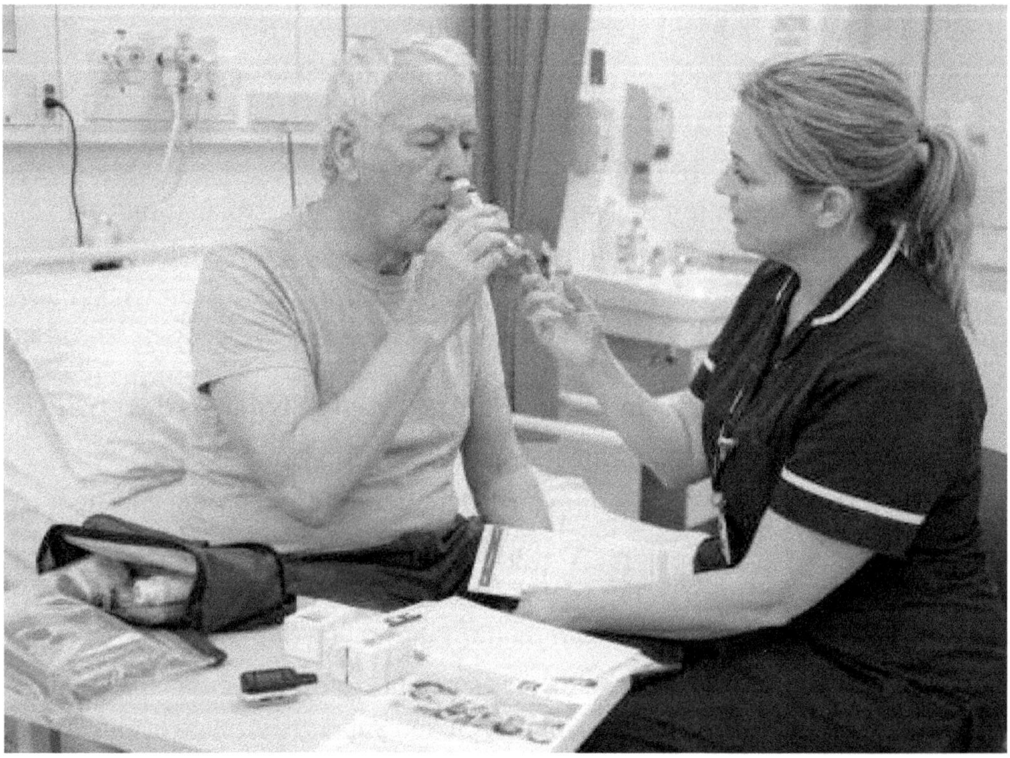

Garnet and Oakley were discharged from the same respiratory ward on the same Thursday, both after exacerbations of chronic obstructive pulmonary disease, both on identical medication, both with follow up requested from their general practices. Garnet was readmitted 11 days later. Oakley was not readmitted that year. Neither difference was explained by disease severity, and both men had been assessed as medically fit for discharge by the same consultant on the same round. What separated them happened in the four hours before each of them left the building, and none of it appeared in either discharge summary.

16.1 The Four Hours

The following are composite cases.

Case A

Garnet's discharge began at eleven in the morning when the decision was made and completed at three when transport arrived. His medications were reconciled by pharmacy. He was given a bag containing two inhalers, one of which was a device he had not used before. A discharge letter was generated requesting that his practice review him within two weeks. Nobody watched him use the new device. His wife collected him and was not spoken to. He was breathless walking to the car and nobody recorded it.

Case B

Oakley's discharge took the same four hours. A nurse asked him to demonstrate both inhalers and found an error in the new one, which she corrected and rechecked twice. She walked with him to the ward door and recorded that he desaturated to 88 percent and needed to stop once. She telephoned his practice rather than relying on the letter and a review was booked for the following Tuesday. She spent ten minutes with his daughter covering what a deterioration would look like and what to do about it. She referred him to pulmonary rehabilitation.

The medical care was identical. The difference was entirely in what was verified rather than issued, and it took one nurse approximately 35 additional minutes.

16.2 What Actually Separated Them

Four things distinguished Oakley's discharge and each maps onto a documented failure mode.

Technique was verified rather than assumed. Chapter 5 established that a documented technique check and a watched demonstration are different events, and that a patient handed an unfamiliar device may receive no drug from it at all.

Function was measured at the point of leaving. A saturation recorded while sitting in a chair at ten in the morning describes a patient who is about to walk to a car, climb stairs at home, and manage a bathroom. Walking the patient before discharge takes four minutes and is the closest thing available to a test of whether the discharge will hold.

Follow up was arranged rather than requested. A letter asking a practice to review a patient is a request that enters a queue. A booked appointment is an arrangement. The distinction is measurable and it is the point at which most discharge plans quietly fail.

And the carer was included. The person who will notice the deterioration first is usually not the patient, and a carer who has been told what to look for and what to do is an early warning system that costs ten minutes to install.

> **Teaching Point:** *Ask yourself one question before any respiratory discharge, which is what has been verified rather than issued. Medicines are issued. Letters are issued. Technique, function, understanding, and follow up have to be verified, and only the second list predicts readmission.*

16.3 The Discharge Bundle

A respiratory discharge that holds contains six elements, and none of them requires a prescriber.

Medicines reconciled, with the patient understanding which are new, which have stopped, and which are for rescue use. Patients discharged after an exacerbation frequently arrive home with both their old and new inhalers and no clear idea which to use, which is the same problem described in Chapter 6 in a different setting.

Technique demonstrated back by the patient, on the actual devices going home, more than once.

A written self management plan that names the patient's own medicines and doses, describes what a deterioration looks like for them, and states what to do and at what point to seek help.

Function assessed on movement, with a specific record of what the patient managed.

Follow up booked and confirmed, with direct contact to the community team where the patient is complex.

And the carer briefed, with explicit escalation criteria.

16.4 Rescue Plans and Rescue Packs

Self management plans work when they are specific and fail when they are generic.

A plan that advises the patient to seek help if they feel worse has restated the problem. A plan that says what worse means for this individual, in terms of their own baseline sputum, their own walking distance, and their own inhaler use, gives them a threshold they can actually apply. Chapter 11 made the same point about sputum baselines and it applies to every condition in this book.

Rescue packs of antibiotics and corticosteroids held at home are used in some services for selected patients. They shorten the interval between deterioration and treatment, and they carry the risk of being used inappropriately or too late. The determinant is whether the patient has been taught when to start them and, critically, that starting them is not a substitute for seeking review. A patient who takes a rescue pack and then waits five days to see whether it works has used the pack to delay rather than to accelerate care.

Patients also need to know what the plan does not cover. A written plan that addresses infective deterioration does not address a sudden severe episode, and a patient needs to know which situations require an ambulance rather than a phone call.

16.5 The Patients Who Need More Than a Plan

Some patients cannot be discharged safely on a standard bundle, and identifying them is a nursing judgment made from the bedside rather than from the notes.

Three groups recur. Patients whose function has not returned to their pre admission baseline, who are being discharged to a home that was already marginal for the person they were a fortnight ago. Patients living alone with no one to notice deterioration, for whom the carer element of the bundle simply does not exist. And patients on their third or fourth admission in a year, for whom the discharge plan has now demonstrably failed several times and repeating it is unlikely to produce a different result.

For the first group, the question is occupational therapy and social assessment rather than medicine, and it needs raising early rather than on the morning of discharge, because it is the commonest cause of a delayed discharge and the commonest thing to be raised too late.

For the second, community respiratory team involvement, telephone follow up, or a virtual ward where one exists substitutes for the absent observer.

For the third group, the honest conversation is a different one. A patient admitted repeatedly with advancing disease is a patient for whom advance care planning is appropriate, and Chapter 10 established that these conversations go better when they begin during a period of relative stability rather than during a crisis. A discharge after a fourth admission is one of the few moments when the trajectory is visible to the patient as well as to the team.

16.6 Home Oxygen and What Patients Discover

Home oxygen is assessed and prescribed by a specialist service against defined criteria, and the ward nurse's role is to identify candidates, prepare patients, and correct misunderstandings.

The most common misunderstanding is the one Chapter 13 addressed, which is that oxygen relieves breathlessness. Patients frequently expect home oxygen to make them feel better and are disappointed when it does not, because long term oxygen therapy is prescribed for survival benefit in chronic hypoxaemia rather than for symptom relief. Setting that expectation before assessment prevents a great deal of subsequent dissatisfaction.

The practical realities are ones patients discover after installation rather than before. Concentrators are noisy and increase electricity costs, for which reimbursement arrangements exist and are frequently not explained. Tubing across a floor is a fall hazard in exactly the population least able to tolerate a fall. Ambulatory cylinders are heavier than people expect.

Fire risk requires a direct conversation rather than a leaflet. Smoking near oxygen causes severe burns and deaths every year. The conversation needs to happen with the patient and with everybody in the household, and it needs to be specific rather than general, because a patient who has been told oxygen is flammable may not connect that with a visitor lighting a cigarette in the next room.

16.7 The Conversations With a Window

Two discharge conversations work far better at this moment than at any other, and both are routinely deferred to a clinic the patient may not attend.

Pulmonary rehabilitation referral is best made while the patient is still in the bed that the exacerbation put them in. The connection between the admission and the offer is visible at that point and becomes abstract within a fortnight. The commonest reason for refusal, as Chapter 13 described, is a belief that becoming breathless during exercise is dangerous, and addressing that belief directly converts more referrals than any amount of describing the programme.

Smoking cessation has a similar window and requires a different tone. A patient recovering from an exacerbation knows perfectly well that smoking is implicated, has usually been told so repeatedly, and has frequently been told so in a way that produced shame rather than change. What works better is to ask whether they have thought about stopping, to offer the pharmacological and behavioural support that exists, and to make the referral. Advice alone performs poorly. Advice plus pharmacotherapy plus behavioural support performs considerably better, and the difference is a referral rather than a conversation.

Neither of these should be delivered on the morning of discharge alongside six other things. Both work better on the day before, when the patient is well enough to think and not yet occupied with going home.

16.8 The Handover That Was Not Read

The following account is a composite, with details changed for anonymity.

Wren, whose first months on a respiratory ward opened Chapter 1, had by this point been qualified for four years and had become the person her ward asked about discharges.

She had reached that position through an uncomfortable route. She had audited the readmissions from her own ward over three months and found that a substantial proportion had a discharge letter requesting general practice follow up and no evidence that any follow up had occurred. The letters had been sent. Nothing had been arranged.

Her first solution was a better letter. She redesigned the discharge summary to highlight the follow up request at the top, and readmission rates did not change, because the problem was never that the request was hard to find. It was that a request is not an appointment.

What worked was telephoning. For patients meeting agreed criteria, a nurse rang the practice before discharge and a review was booked while the patient was still on the ward. This took approximately eight minutes per patient and it was, she said, the single most useful change she had made in four years.

She was clear about its fragility. The practice depended on there being enough staff to make the calls, it lapsed during periods of short staffing, and it had not been written into any policy. When she moved to a different post it continued for a few months and then stopped. She described this without much surprise, having by then watched the same pattern with the baseline question in Chapter 4.

Teaching points:

A discharge letter transfers information and does not transfer responsibility, and the distinction is where most follow up plans fail.

An improvement that depends on individual effort rather than on a system will not survive the person who introduced it, which is an argument for writing things into policy rather than doing them well.

Settling the Account

Three things in this chapter are supported well enough to act on without hesitation. Verified inhaler technique on the actual device going home changes whether treatment is delivered at all. Booked follow up outperforms requested follow up, and the difference is not marginal. And a briefed carer with explicit escalation criteria detects deterioration earlier than the patient does.

Two things are reasonable and less certain. Walking a patient before discharge and recording what happened is obviously more informative than a resting saturation, and it has not been established that it changes readmission rates. Rescue packs shorten time to treatment for some patients and are used inappropriately by others, and which effect dominates depends on selection and teaching in ways that are difficult to specify from a ward.

One thing in this chapter is uncomfortable and should be stated plainly. Almost every improvement described here was achieved by an individual nurse doing something extra that was not in any policy, and in both documented instances it stopped when that nurse left. Briar's baseline question in Chapter 4 and Wren's telephone calls in section 16.8 were effective and neither survived. That is not a story about exceptional individuals. It is a description of how respiratory nursing improvement usually works and usually fails.

The practical implication is that the most durable thing a nurse can do with the content of this book is not to practise it well. It is to get it written down somewhere that outlives her, which is a slower, duller, and considerably more consequential piece of work than any single discharge.

Chapter 16 Review Questions

1. Which discharge action most reliably ensures that follow up occurs?

A) A discharge letter with the follow up request highlighted

B) A booked and confirmed appointment, with direct contact to the community team where appropriate

C) Advising the patient to contact their practice on discharge

D) Providing a copy of the discharge summary to the patient

Answer: B. A request enters a queue. An arrangement is an appointment. This distinction accounts for a substantial share of failed discharge plans.

2. A patient is discharged with a new inhaler device they have not used before. What is the minimum acceptable standard before discharge?

A) Written information about the device is provided

B) The patient states that they understand how to use it

C) The patient demonstrates correct technique on the actual device, on more than one occasion

D) Technique will be checked at the follow up appointment

Answer: C. A stated understanding and a demonstrated technique are different events. A patient discharged with a device they cannot use is receiving no treatment from it.

3. What is the principal purpose of long term oxygen therapy in chronic hypoxaemia?

A) Relief of breathlessness

B) Survival benefit in appropriately selected hypoxaemic patients

C) Improvement in exercise tolerance

D) Reduction in exacerbation frequency

Answer: B. Patients frequently expect symptomatic relief and are disappointed. Setting this expectation before assessment prevents dissatisfaction and inappropriate use.

Afterword

Go back to the five questions in the preface and answer them again.

Most readers who do this find the same pattern. The oxygen question and the blood gas question are now easy, because both have a fixed sequence and sequences survive. The inhaler question is answered differently, and usually with less confidence than the first time, which is the correct direction of travel. The ventilation question is answered with more caution and more precision. And the question about what to say to a frightened patient is answered with a sentence rather than a principle, which is the whole of the difference.

The patient at the end of the bed in the introduction was drowsy at 89 percent with no oxygen prescription. The answer is now unremarkable. He is at risk of hypercapnic respiratory failure, his target range is probably 88 to 92 percent, the drowsiness is the finding that matters far more than the saturation, and the absence of a prescription is a clinical problem rather than a paperwork one. He needs a blood gas and he needs it now, and the sentence that will produce one describes what has changed rather than what the number is.

That answer took sixteen chapters to make obvious. It should have taken a shift.

What to Do With This Next

Three things, in order of how much they will cost you.

The cheapest is to keep checking currency. Everything clinical in this book is dated in the text for one reason, which is that it will go out of date. The asthma position changed in 2024. The chronic obstructive disease framework changed in 2023. The oxygen guidance has held since 2017 and will not hold forever. Four sources will keep you current, and reading a guideline update properly takes about twenty minutes if you go straight to the summary of recommendations and the section describing what has changed since the previous version.

The second is to teach it. Fifteen minutes at a handover, on one topic, with one thing to practise. Inhaler critical errors works well because the self test produces a result people remember. Blood gases in four questions works well because it is short enough to finish. Ventilation set up works well because most staff have never been shown it slowly. Teaching a thing is also the most reliable way of discovering which parts of it you do not actually understand, which is uncomfortable and useful in that order.

The third is the expensive one, and it is the argument this book has kept returning to.

Briar asked every patient what they had been able to do a week ago, and it worked, and it stopped when she moved wards. Wren telephoned practices to book follow up appointments, and it worked, and it stopped when she left. Joss learned to watch a patient's inhaler technique in silence, from nobody in particular, and it is not written down anywhere. Xael wrote up night conversations about dying that he had no confidence anybody read. Vesper learned the most important thing she knows about being with dying patients from a single remark by one colleague.

Every one of those is a real improvement in patient care that depended entirely on one person and did not survive them. That is not a story about heroic individuals and it is not a criticism of the units involved. It is the ordinary mechanism by which good respiratory nursing gets lost, repeatedly, and it is why the same national reports keep finding the same things a decade apart.

So the third thing is the dull one. Write it into something. A checklist, a proforma, an induction pack, a line in a local policy, a standing item on a handover sheet. It is slower than doing the thing well yourself, it produces no visible result on any given shift, and it is the only version of this that outlasts you.

A Closing Note on Limits

This book has been direct about clinical decisions because vagueness is not safer, and it has been repetitive about one boundary for the same reason.

You are working within a registration, a competency framework, and a local policy. This book explains what is happening and why so that you can recognise it, describe it accurately, and escalate it credibly. It does not extend what you are permitted to do, and there is no situation described in these pages where understanding the physiology better is a substitute for calling somebody who can act.

The nurses who manage respiratory patients best are not the ones who intervene most. They are the ones who notice earliest, describe most precisely, and ask most specifically. Everything in the preceding sixteen chapters is in service of those three things.

References

Bolton, C. E., Bevan-Smith, E. F., Blakey, J. D., Crowe, P., Elkin, S. L., Garrod, R., Greening, N. J., Heslop, K., Hull, J. H., Man, W. D.-C., Morgan, M. D., Proud, D., Roberts, C. M., Sewell, L., Singh, S. J., Walker, P. P., & Walmsley, S. (2013). British Thoracic Society guideline on pulmonary rehabilitation in adults. Thorax, 68(Suppl 2), ii1-ii30. https://doi.org/10.1136/thoraxjnl-2013-203808

British Thoracic Society, National Institute for Health and Care Excellence, & Scottish Intercollegiate Guidelines Network. (2024). Asthma: Diagnosis, monitoring and chronic asthma management (NICE guideline NG245). National Institute for Health and Care Excellence. https://www.nice.org.uk/guidance/ng245

British Thoracic Society, National Institute for Health and Care Excellence, & Scottish Intercollegiate Guidelines Network. (2025). BTS/NICE/SIGN joint guideline on asthma: Diagnosis, monitoring and chronic asthma management (November 2024). Summary of recommendations. Thorax. https://doi.org/10.1136/thorax-2024-222910

Chu, D. K., Kim, L. H., Young, P. J., Zamiri, N., Almenawer, S. A., Jaeschke, R., Szczeklik, W., Schunemann, H. J., Neary, J. D., & Alhazzani, W. (2018). Mortality and morbidity in acutely ill adults treated with liberal versus conservative oxygen therapy (IOTA): A systematic review and meta-analysis. The Lancet, 391(10131), 1693-1705. https://doi.org/10.1016/S0140-6736(18)30479-3

Davidson, A. C., Banham, S., Elliott, M., Kennedy, D., Gelder, C., Glossop, A., Church, A. C., Creagh-Brown, B., Dodd, J. W., Felton, T., Foex, B., Mansfield, L., McDonnell, L., Parker, R., Patterson, C. M., Sovani, M., & Thomas, L. (2016). BTS/ICS guideline for the ventilatory management of acute hypercapnic respiratory failure in adults. Thorax, 71(Suppl 2), ii1-ii35. https://doi.org/10.1136/thoraxjnl-2015-208209

Davies, M., Allen, M., Bentley, A., Bourke, S. C., Creagh-Brown, B., D'Oliveiro, R., Glossop, A., Gray, A., Jacobs, P., Mahadeva, R., Moses, R., & Setchfield, I. (2018). British Thoracic Society Quality Standards for acute non-invasive ventilation in adults. BMJ Open Respiratory Research, 5(1), e000283. https://doi.org/10.1136/bmjresp-2018-000283

Galbraith, S., Fagan, P., Perkins, P., Lynch, A., & Booth, S. (2010). Does the use of a handheld fan improve chronic dyspnea? A randomized, controlled, crossover trial. Journal of Pain and Symptom Management, 39(5), 831-838. https://doi.org/10.1016/j.jpainsymman.2009.09.024

Global Initiative for Chronic Obstructive Lung Disease. (2025). Global strategy for the prevention, diagnosis and management of chronic obstructive pulmonary disease: 2025 report. https://goldcopd.org

Hill, A. T., Sullivan, A. L., Chalmers, J. D., De Soyza, A., Elborn, J. S., Floto, R. A., Grillo, L., Gruffydd-Jones, K., Harvey, A., Haworth, C. S., Hiscocks, E., Hurst, J. R., Johnson, C., Kelleher, W. P., Bedi, P., Payne, K., Saleh, H., Screaton, N. J., Smith, M., ... Loebinger, M. R. (2019). British Thoracic Society guideline for bronchiectasis in adults. Thorax, 74(Suppl 1), 1-69. https://doi.org/10.1136/thoraxjnl-2018-212463

Johnston, K. N., Young, M., Kay, D., Booth, S., Spathis, A., & Williams, M. T. (2020). Attitude change and increased confidence with management of chronic breathlessness following a health professional training workshop: A survey evaluation. BMC Medical Education, 20(1), 90. https://doi.org/10.1186/s12909-020-02006-7

McGrath, B. A., Bates, L., Atkinson, D., & Moore, J. A. (2012). Multidisciplinary guidelines for the management of tracheostomy and laryngectomy airway emergencies. Anaesthesia, 67(9), 1025-1041. https://doi.org/10.1111/j.1365-2044.2012.07217.x

Medicines and Healthcare products Regulatory Agency. (2025, April). Short-acting beta-2 agonists (salbutamol, terbutaline): Reminder of the risks from overuse in asthma and to be aware of changes in SABA prescribing guidelines. Drug Safety Update. https://www.gov.uk/drug-safety-update

National Confidential Enquiry into Patient Outcome and Death. (2017). Inspiring change: A review of the quality of care provided to patients receiving acute non-invasive ventilation. NCEPOD. https://www.ncepod.org.uk/2017niv.html

National Institute for Health and Care Excellence. (2019). Chronic obstructive pulmonary disease in over 16s: Diagnosis and management (NICE guideline NG115). https://www.nice.org.uk/guidance/ng115

O'Driscoll, B. R., Howard, L. S., Earis, J., & Mak, V. (2017). BTS guideline for oxygen use in adults in healthcare and emergency settings. Thorax, 72(Suppl 1), ii1-ii90. https://doi.org/10.1136/thoraxjnl-2016-209729

Roberts, M. E., Rahman, N. M., Maskell, N. A., Bibby, A. C., Blyth, K. G., Corcoran, J. P., Edey, A., Evison, M., de Fonseka, D., Hallifax, R., Harden, S., Lawrie, I., Lim, E., McCracken, D., Mercer, R., Mishra, E. K., Nicholson, A. G., Noorzad, F., Opstad, K. S., ... Walker, S. (2023). British Thoracic Society guideline for pleural disease. Thorax, 78(11), 1143-1156. https://doi.org/10.1136/thorax-2023-220304

Royal College of Physicians. (2014). Why asthma still kills: The National Review of Asthma Deaths (NRAD) confidential enquiry report. Royal College of Physicians. https://www.rcp.ac.uk/improving-care/resources/why-asthma-still-kills/

Russell, A. M., Lines, S., Olive, S., Murphy, A., Hocking, J., Newell, K., Morris, H., Harris, E., Dixon, C., Agnew, S., & Burge, G. (2018). Contemporary challenges for specialist nursing in interstitial lung disease. Breathe, 14(1), 36-43. https://doi.org/10.1183/20734735.014917

Spathis, A., Booth, S., Moffat, C., Hurst, R., Ryan, R., Chin, C., & Burkin, J. (2017). The Breathing, Thinking, Functioning clinical model: A proposal to facilitate evidence-based breathlessness management in chronic respiratory disease. npj Primary Care Respiratory Medicine, 27, 27. https://doi.org/10.1038/s41533-017-0024-z

Spathis, A., Burkin, J., Moffat, C., Tuffnell, R., Barclay, S., Mant, J., & Booth, S. (2021). Cutting through complexity: The Breathing, Thinking, Functioning clinical model is an educational tool that facilitates chronic breathlessness management. npj Primary Care Respiratory Medicine, 31, 25. https://doi.org/10.1038/s41533-021-00237-9

Swami, V., Cho, J.-G., Smith, T., Wheatley, J., & Roberts, M. (2021). Confidence of nurses with inhaler device education and competency of device use in a specialised respiratory inpatient unit. Chronic Respiratory Disease, 18, 14799731211002241. https://doi.org/10.1177/14799731211002241

www.ingramcontent.com/pod-product-compliance
Lightning Source LLC
LaVergne TN
LVHW081739071126
851857LV00041B/1794